Lay Aside the Weight

Lay Aside the Weight

Taking Control of It Before
It Takes Control of You!

by

Bishop T. D. Jakes

ALBURY PUBLISHING
Tulsa, Oklahoma

Fourth Printing

Contents

Dedication

I would like to dedicate this book to my wife Serita, who joined me in the change and whose encouragement has always enabled me to achieve my goals.

I also want to dedicate this book to my sister Jacqueline, whose tremendous weight loss challenged and convicted me. Thank you for warning me, caring for my health, and silently supporting my dreams.

Lastly, I want to dedicate this to all who have tried and wrestled, succeeded, and failed. I have not written to preach to you, but to encourage you. We must help one another. Keep praying for me as I fight my giants, and I will continue to pray for you. God knows that life is full of giants. But remember: All things are possible to him who believes.

Wherefore seeing we also are compassed about
with so great a cloud of witnesses,
let us lay aside every weight,
and the sin which doth so easily beset us,
and let us run with patience
the race that is set before us,
looking unto Jesus
the author and finisher of our faith.

Hebrews 12:1,2

chapter 1

Hey Giant! Who You Callin' Fat?

Summer doesn't scare me anymore.

Of all the intimidating things in the world, who would think that the blaring, hot, sun-drenched beaches would cause a person to cower? Normally, walking hand-in-hand in the warm, evening breeze or picnics in the park would not be frightening. But to a few of us, summer was a time that underscored our lack of discipline in vivid terms. Sunshine exposed the sad rewards of overindulgence.

Heavily clad in vain cover-ups, we knew that the high summer temperatures might cause us to have a heat stroke! That might sound strange, but many people will understand what I mean. I can remember being concerned when my friends would slip out of their sweaters and sweat pants into their summer T-shirts and shorts to enjoy the outdoor fun.

Why did that concern a fit-looking fellow like me? I am glad you asked. I guess it was the same reason that makes women go on crash diets when they realize they are going to the beach. It was the heart-wrenching, pulse-racing panic that comes when you realize you are going to be the only one lying on the beach who attracts whale watchers.

It was the feeling of regret that comes on you when you walk past a mirror and catch a side view of what your wife must see all the time. I had more dimples than Shirley Temple — but mine were not on my face! They were in strange places like my back and neck and other unmentionable locations.

Winter is an overweight person's best friend. The coats, scarves, sweaters, and jackets benefit them, even if it isn't cold. A person can wear a lighter weight coat and camouflage the rounded terrain of his bulbous silhouette. Additionally helpful is the new trend that the youth are wearing in over-sized clothes. I mean, it seems fashionable to them to look at least three sizes larger than they are. I guess I thought I could wear these tent like garments and make a fashion statement. It was a statement that was abbreviated by the approaching warmth of summer.

> Should you happen to notice that another person is extremely tall or overweight, eats too much or declines convivial drinks, has red hair or goes about in a wheelchair, ought to get married or ought not to be pregnant — see if you can refrain from bringing these astonishing observations to that person's attention.
>
> — Judith Martin, "Miss Manners"

Yes, summer is the time when trees begin to dress themselves with green leaves and extended branches. It is the time when the smell of honeysuckle fills the air and geese make their yearly pilgrimage back to the warmth of climates they forsook for a few months to avoid the cold blight of winter's icy finger.

Even the tinkling sound of children's laughter could not woo me into a delightful mood as I suddenly found myself envious of men who could at least walk around dressed for the weather without looking like a fall catalog for J. C. Penney's. As long pants gave way to shorts and long sleeves were sliced in half, I shuddered.

Every year I watched the parading of my peers, who were the same age as me, shed themselves of the cumbersome entanglements of winter garb and head for the streets, smiling in the breeze. They dressed in the simple garments that are associated with the frivolity of the festive summer weather.

I do not think I was depressed or insecure to the degree that I was engrossed with the issue, but I must admit that I avoided taking off my coat if at all possible. I smile even thinking about it now. I know I wouldn't have admitted it, but my jacket was to me what Linus' blanket was to him. You remember Linus, the character created by Charles Schultz in the Charlie Brown comic strip? Linus never went anywhere without his blanket, and I never went anywhere without my coat! When I think about it, I realize that the coat might have been more conspicuous than the weight. But at that time, I thought it was at least more attractive.

Now, after one year of taking control of my health and shedding nearly 100 pounds, I must admit I feel a lot better without the weight — and without the coat! Although I still might not want to pose for a bathing suit commercial, I do feel pleased to have accomplished what was at one time a bit like fighting a Goliath in my life.

I know that it is not the size of the ship that makes the motion of the ocean, but I felt like the Titanic in the summer. However, I do not think I would have gained the courage to confront my weight without the devil attacking my health. When he tried to attack me physically I said, "All right, that's it!"

Everyone has a breaking point. I don't know what yours is, but I found mine. I remember when another customer at a restaurant handed me a brochure on a weight-loss program as I was leaving. I was so angry when I saw what it was, I wanted to start a fight. I nearly forgot my ministry, my reputation, and everything else. I wanted to slug the customer. I can see the papers now: "*Nationally renowned evangelist lays hands on customer in restaurant!*"

I was furious that these vitamin-selling health addicts would infringe upon my privacy like tacky evangelists, passing out their health tracts and witnessing to the obese. What was worse, the customer in question looked about as fit as a stuffed bell pepper in a school lunch line. I wanted to say, "Look at the way you are pouring over your shoes!"

I am sure that no one else can decide to confront your weight but you. All who try will only insult you and estrange themselves from you. Sometimes you wonder if these no-tact evangelist-type program promoters' real motivation is not so much the rehabilitation of the obese, as it is the chance to sell some new product. They fail to understand that the real product with which we need to face this challenge — or any challenge — isn't in a bottle. It is in the Bible! I have found no greater motivational tool anywhere than this guide to truth which most Christians read everyday.

The fads that come to us from someone else's opinion about what is attractive can cause us pain. We cannot allow the ideas of others to determine how we feel about ourselves. It is that sort of public empowerment that leads to anorexia and other eating disorders. Faddish ideas cause us to feel that no loss is ever great enough. We cannot receive our cues from the opinion of others, because life will always afford us at least one or two critics, no matter what we do.

The battle over weight is a giant that has to be fought because *you* are tired of it and *you* want a change. It has to be fought by you, for you, and for those who love you as you are. They do not want to lose you to this war with the giant that threatens to increase within you!

Man, oh man, is it ever a war! For some of us, the fight is more difficult than for others. Some of our struggle may be our genetics, and some of it is our cultures. Many of us who are prone to obesity may not be overeaters but we may be undereducated to the information needed to make better choices.

It has been said that knowledge is power, and it really is. We will talk more about it later, but the Bible says, "My people perish for the lack of knowledge," and it is true. (See Hosea 4:6.) It is true about finances, it is true about moral weakness, and it is even true about living healthy lives. This book is written to give you the tools you need to fight the good fight of faith. That faith comes by hearing and hearing by the Word of God.

> Happy is the man that findeth wisdom, and the man that getteth understanding... Length of days is in her right hand; and in her left hand riches and honour.
>
> Proverbs 3:13,16

I am not about to put down my Bible, grab my tennis shoes, and spend the rest of my life doing exercise videos. In fact, I wouldn't even tackle this rather personal issue of sharing my testimony about losing weight if there were not so many people asking the same questions.

The number one question whispered to me in airports across America is, "How did you do it?" Many people who ask seemingly have no weight problem, but they are concerned about living healthier lives and maximizing their strength for the Master's use.

My story doesn't begin with me. It begins with my father and perhaps with his father before him. My grandfather, who was also called T. D., died at an early age. He died before I was born and before my father was an adult. Isn't it strange that my father also died before completing his assignment with his children? I did not know all the details surrounding my grandfather's death, but I was watching front and center when my father made his exit from this world.

My father, Ernest L. Jakes Sr., was a rather robust, gregarious kind of fellow who was of large stature. I can still see him in my mind. I catch glimpses of him in my mirror, as I look a lot like him.

By the time he was about forty, he had built a rather successful business in Charleston. He had taken a mop and a bucket and turned it into a janitorial company. In its zenith, the company had fifty employees. For a man of color to build a successful company at that time was quite a feat. He was proud of it and deeply involved with his work. Today we would call him a workaholic. Nevertheless, he didn't stop until a job was done.

He had taken a physical to do some work for a prestigious company in West Virginia when they discovered that his blood pressure was very, very high. It was approximately 190 over 150. We did not know how long it had been elevated, but as I look back, it had probably been high for quite awhile. I assume that, because they recommended he go immediately to Cleveland Clinic. There, they discovered that his blood pressure had hopelessly scarred his kidneys and he had gone into renal failure.

Little did I know that their diagnosis would also effect my life, as well as his, forever.

What I did know was that my father, who already seemed light-headed and had started to stagger when he walked, was never going to be the same again. He was in the clinic for weeks, and when he did come home he was weak and weary and had lost a lot of weight. Sadly, he lost the weight too late.

My father went down to 130 pounds. He looked like a skeleton and he never again was the man I used to think of as Hercules. His broad shoulders and strong arms became listless, poorly animated objects that only hinted at being recognizable limbs.

He was gone in a flash — not dead, not yet anyway — but he was gone. The vibrance, the life, the strength, and the stamina was gone from him. I still remember thinking how unfair it seemed. He had finally built his dream house and had established his company, but now he was so sick he couldn't enjoy it.

For the next eight years he would be exiled to live in a body that was in total rebellion to his will. He would eat food that tasted like cardboard and drink cranberry juice by the gallon. In spite of being dialyzed twice a week and following all the instructions the doctors prescribed, he was a mere shadow of the man whose arms had previously looked like tree limbs.

My daddy was sick, and he never recovered. I traded my toys, my sports activities, and my childhood for hospital waiting rooms with their faint smell of formaldehyde, which was used to wash the membranes of the kidney dialysis machines.

I waved good-bye to my childhood and hello to responsibility. I waved good-bye to my friends, then after a long hard discouraging fight, I stood staring down into a red clay hole in Waynesboro, Mississippi, and waved good-bye to my father. We had lost the fight.

I spent eight years fighting his death, and the next eight years trying to accept it. But what can one do with the dead except learn to accept what none of us can change? We can accept it and learn from it, and so I did. I learned from what his death taught me. I learned to survive, to endure, and to continue.

Twenty-two years later, I found myself at a similar age fighting a similar challenge. It was as if Satan had left our family for a season and then returned for the next generation. The devil thought he was going to get a fresh harvest of Jakes' blood. I was at the same stage and the same age as my father when he fell prey.

There I was ministering in Washington, DC, when I knew that something was wrong. Now there is a difference between being sick and being tired. And there was no time to be insulted this time. No time for denial either. Goliath was coming and only I, alone, could fight him off.

I had not noticed that being driven to reach the world for Jesus had caused me to ignore my own well-being. I couldn't tell you when I had gained so much weight. I must have known it. I had bought all new clothes to accommodate it.

> In order to be free from the senseless suffering that is produced by being physically unfit, a person must suffer in another way, but it is a type of suffering that leads to victory and ultimately brings an end to suffering.
>
> — Joyce Meyer

I was wearing a size 40 extra-long suit when I married my wife. Then one day I blinked and found myself wearing a 56 extra-long suit. I don't know which sweet potato pie did that to me. I can't point to the banana pudding that attacked me. Maybe it was that midnight fried chicken extravaganza that caused me to blossom. All I know is that I looked around and the scales in hotels could no longer document my weight gain. I was 338 pounds and still going.

I told myself it didn't matter. I thought all that really counted was being available to God for His use. Until, while I was preaching one day, I noticed that my feet were swelling. I thought it was the traveling, but it wasn't. My wife pressed the swelling that had started up my legs and her fingerprint left its mark in my flesh. I had not seen anything like that since I had washed my dad's legs.

Well, can you believe that? Satan could have at least used a new demon. But no, he used that same demon that attacked my dad. It was then that I realized every man has got to fight his father's enemy — in one form or another. We all must fight the spirits that have been assigned to our families.

Even physicians now ask questions about the medical history of your parents. They do it because they know to be forewarned is to be forearmed. They ask about your grandparents' illnesses, because they know certain families are more susceptible to certain afflictions. You might escape it in your youth as I did. I never had any trace of a problem until recently, but time brings about a change.

I began to evaluate the Scriptures and noticed that the same thing that is true with the physical man is also true with the spiritual man. King David wrestled with lust. He had an ongoing battle with his sexuality. He was anointed, but he was also sensual and prone to eroticism.

David's interlude with Bathsheba was just the tip of the iceberg. He was a man of great passion. His son Abnon wrestled with his father's tendency to a lustful disposition and raped his sister. His son Solomon had 700 wives and 300 concubines who turned his heart away from God. Wonder where he got that tendency from?

Jacob was as deceitful as his mother Rebecca had been. They were both sneaky and cunning, deceiving even those whom they supposedly loved. His Uncle Laban was a con artist also. It seemed that treachery ran in the family.

If you can evaluate what sickness runs in your family, you can head off certain attacks, or at least better position yourself to fight them. I had a significant understanding of the spirit assigned to attack me from experiencing the death of my father.

To be equipped for the fight, you have to be prepared for your enemy. He has a certain strategy that he thinks he can use on you. He tried it on me, but I decided to live. I have shed nearly 100 pounds at this writing. Beyond any cosmetic reasons for losing weight, there is one reason that extends beyond all other reasons: Life.

As we get older our hearts take a beating hauling around extra weight equivalent to carrying another person. My ten-year-old daughter doesn't quite weigh 100 pounds. But it was like I was carrying her around on my body and on my heart. So I decided to lay aside the weight. At least my father's death would make some sense if it helped to warn me to get back to my correct weight before it was too late.

I looked at my five children and thought of how I grew up sitting in waiting rooms impatient to hear a word about my father. I thought about the games I didn't get to see and the achievements my dad never got to witness. I decided that I wanted more for my family than what I had already endured.

As a result I began to build up my spirit to take on the giant of my life. My enemy had, like Goliath, killed others before me. He was armed with a long resumé of all the reasons why he could not be slain. But I decided: Win, loose, sink, or swim, there is one thing that is certain. We are going to fight!

chapter 2

Goliath Was a Small Man, After All

The fat giant lays dormant in the lives of busy people.

Those who are preoccupied with less important issues than their own health soon become slaves to food. They hustle and bustle along, prioritizing other things above themselves. In retrospect, I realize Christians are prime candidates to be attacked by this giant. We are so committed to the cause of ministry to others that we have a tendency to live a martyr's life.

It is quite unconscious, I am sure, but we ministers, business people, moms, and dads all have a tendency to lose our passion for caring for ourselves, since we are so intensely focused on what we are assigned to do. It is a challenging issue to identify, because we have another source from which we derive self-esteem — our work!

When work becomes the passion, food becomes the sedative. We go to food for comfort when we are frustrated or tired. We find solace in the pleasant taste of food at the end of a day. We martyrs are not prone to going out just for the activity. That would be too much like having a life outside of what we do!

We would rather come home, slump down in a chair, and swallow a whole pizza. One pizza has enough fat grams to support us for a month. We could fast for thirty days before we used up the fat in that one meal!

Somewhere, hidden in the temptation of eating the whole hot, spicy, gooey texture of cheeses and crumbled morsels of hamburger, pepperoni, hot peppers, succulent crust, and anchovies (if you are so inclined), lies a demonic spirit with a pitch fork saying, "I am going to swell up in you until your thighs look like the columns on your neighbor's front porch!"

But who can resist the tempter's snare when you have worked hard and had a great day? After all, this is reward time, isn't it? Isn't that what we feel when we get home? At last, I am home where I can relax.

I am hungry, starved, famished. Never mind that I swallowed whole a greasy burger, like the big fish that devoured Jonah. That burger is refusing to be ignored, laying somewhere in my stomach praying and asking God for a chance to preach. About two o'clock in the morning, I really see why that whale coughed up Jonah and Ninevah repented!

It is amazing how long these and other bad habits can lay dormant in you and not attack in an obvious way. And then suddenly you hear the *expansion* of the giant. He laughs as he nudges you further and further down the rack to find the bigger dress or belt size. I told myself that the designers were cutting the suits too small — you know, European cuts and all. Yeah, right! It wasn't the cut of the suit. It was the size of the man.

> Know this for truth, and learn to conquer these: Thy belly first; sloth, luxury, and rage. Do nothing base with others or alone, And, above all, thine own self respect.
>
> — Pythagoras

I knew I should lose some weight, but I had an appointment to go to — and the giant dozed back to sleep. Out of sight, hidden under larger clothes and a few undeserved compliments, all was well with the world, wasn't it? I thought I heard something snore. Never mind, the people need me — got to go.

While we push on and on, we never think about those small granular-sized particles of fat floating inside our cardio-vascular system, smiling, bathing, and dancing like the California Raisins. Imagine sharing your body with those little dancing creatures floating in your blood like too many kids playing in the pool! No wonder we are losing so many talented, gifted people to heart attacks. The California Fat Grams are invading our cardio-vascular highways.

I thought it would be terrible to die at an earlier age than I was meant to die. It would be terrible to lose what I had worked all of my life to see. I would miss my wife, my children, and my ministry coming to fruition. But, I will be honest, it was not the fear of death that gave me the courage to attack the fat that was attacking me. I had lived all of my life getting ready to see Jesus. It wasn't the anxiety of losing my wife and children, though that would be devastating, that invoked my war with weight. The thing that gave me the courage to fight was the fear of getting stuck between two worlds.

I had seen my father stuck in a state of sickness so long that his death, though it was the worst moment of my life, was far less cruel than his constant pain and affliction. All right, I admit it. The man of great faith and power has a half cup of cowardice in his recipe. I was jello, shaking and nervous about getting stuck between life and death. There. I have said it. You know it now. I was plain chicken! The real truth is that every one can relate to the desire to avoid incessant suffering.

I decided, rather than facing the agony my father suffered, I had better do something to alleviate the strain on my body before it turned in a leave of absence and quit on me in the middle of my life. I was blessed in that I believe I caught my enemy before he was fully roused in my life.

Goliath was on his way to consciousness when I decided to pray for a strategy to overcome him. I guess I caught him off guard, because when you have been lax for a long time, it is as if your body doesn't expect you to challenge it. But surprise, surprise, surprise! We attacked at daybreak.

> "Then he [David] took his staff in his hand, chose five smooth stones from the stream, put them in the pouch of his shepherd's bag and, with his sling in his hand, approached the Philistine."
>
> 1 Samuel 17:40 NIV

I abruptly assaulted my lifestyle armed with motivational scriptures that I will share throughout this book. I armed myself with a strong prayer and a picture of the family I would miss seeing if I lost this fight. I punched that fat guy in the mirror right in the kisser! Bam! I hit him with a shock.

I snatched those fat grams right out from under him. I didn't ask for a vote or anything. I just snatched them. When I tell you my old flesh had an attitude, please believe me. For the next three days I went through serious withdrawal. He sent some big fat spirit of depression that said, "If you are not going to get to eat what you want you might as well be dead!"

Flesh fights back. But the Bible teaches us that we are already in a war between the flesh and the spirit. The Scriptures declare that as the outward man perishes, the inward man is renewed from day to day. That outward man really doesn't like to perish, and he doesn't like to be denied. If you do not pray he will not be thwarted. It is far more a spiritual issue than I would have ever thought.

Every day I resist temptation I experience the triumph of spirit over flesh. Flesh sends depression because you have changed your habits. You have denied your flesh, and now he says that food is the joy of your life! He wants you to believe that if you do not eat what you want when you want to eat it, you might as well fall over and croak!

That sounds like a spoiled child having a tantrum — and that is exactly what it is! Your flesh is having a tantrum. I said to myself, "It is written — the devil is a liar!" Ohhh, the devil screams when you use the Word of God against him. I said, "Scream all you want, giant. We are going to fight. It is written, 'Man shall not live by bread alone, but by every word of God'" (Luke 4:4).

I wanted the enemy to know that my source doesn't live in the refrigerator. My source is my God. Besides, I refuse to die over a piece of banana cream pie. When I get to heaven and all the disciples are sharing their testimonies, telling how they laid their lives down on chopping blocks and were beheaded for preaching the Gospel, I don't want to be ashamed. I refuse to be the only set of lard-wrapped hips sitting on a cloud saying, "I was slain by a slab of barbecue ribs!"

Armed with headphones sometimes and videos other times, I started working out on my new treadmill. I purchased one because I knew that where there is no investment, there is no commitment. Maybe you cannot get your own treadmill. If not, get a pair of jogging shoes, join a health club, or play tennis. Whatever works for you — but know that spending guilt money is not the answer if you are not going to use what you bought!

I made a decision that worked for me. I prayed about all of the new weight loss pills. I had some on my dresser, but I wasn't led to use them. The Lord impressed on my heart to use His Word instead. It has far less side effects and it builds one thing up while controlling the other.

The Word builds you up mentally and spiritually while attacking the lethargic part of your lifestyle. Long before they came out with the recent warnings about diet pills, I was led to just trust God for my healing. Weight loss is a healing from misplaced priorities, stress, and allowing others around you to dictate your behavior. Physicians heal with medicine, and perhaps some might need that. I do know that Christians have alterntive methods. I decided to pray and apply the Word.

I will admit that it is easier to fight when you have not already become overwhelmed with a sickness. But, I also believe that as long as there is life, there is hope. It is never too late to change your habits and strengthen your life. There is no need to cry, "Save me! Save me!" while you gobble up Manhattan, stumbling around the refrigerator like King Kong in one of those old movies.

The Bible says in James 2:17 that faith without works is dead, being alone. It is better to start on your own than it is to be coerced into it while you are seriously ill. Still, I must tell you that the stirring of the giant was an extreme motivation to kill him quickly.

I used to watch movies with my wife — you know, the kind where there is an assailant in the house and the husband is trying to fight him off. You can always see the woman in the corner screaming. That is the first mistake. I told my wife, "If you ever see me fighting to save our lives and the guy is stomping me into the dirt, don't just scream. Grab a lamp and take the kingdom by force!"

As a child my family's menu consisted of two choices; take it, or leave it.

— Buddy Hackett

I know that sounds humorous, but I say that because if you are married you have to fight enemies together. If you can get your companion to fight the giant with you, it is for your good. Most guys eat whatever their wives put in front of them anyway. Also, it is easier for a lady to lose weight if she doesn't have to make apple strudel every morning for King Daddy Bear over there! When there is agreement in the family, it is easier. But if you have to go it alone, please do it. It is worth the fight.

The other thing that drives me crazy in those old films is when the couple finally have the criminal down and they walk away without insuring he doesn't get up again. I say, "When you have him down, make sure he doesn't get up again!" In that same way, when you get the courage to defend yourself and change your lifestyle, don't play around with it. Go all the way. Kill that giant. Don't scold him or slap his hands. Kill him! Always remember: Whatever enemy you do not destroy in your life will ultimately destroy you.

My wife and I fought the same giant, but we fought in different ways. I chose to use more exercise and have a broader food base. She chose less exercise with a narrow food base. It is simple. If you take more liberty in the kitchen, you have to pay your dues in the gym. She chose to exercise, but not to go overboard in the gym. Instead she was very disciplined in her eating habits.

Well, I cheated and still do from time to time. But I am careful about what excesses I take. When I do, I pay for it in the morning on the treadmill. I can tell you one thing, when you realize how much you have to walk to pay for a piece of pie, it will turn you against cheating!

Since this is not a diet, but a behavioral modification you are going to maintain permanently, you have to design it to accommodate your greatest strengths. There is a program that will personally accommodate your lifestyle and your personality.

Choose exercises you enjoy. If there are none that you enjoy, choose to do them in places you enjoy. Maybe walking in the park might be better for you than walking on a treadmill. Perhaps watching an action movie will make the treadmill more exciting. Try walking with people who want to talk to you. Tell them to hang up the phone and meet you in the park.

Avoid having fellowship or counseling over food. The more engrossed you get in the conversation, the more you eat. Disassociate eating from fellowship. Many times we eat subconsciously because we do it while we are doing something else. In that same way, you can exercise unconsciously if you do it while you are being distracted by something else.

I encourage you to remember that giants do die. David vanquished Goliath by refusing to be intimidated. The giant had a long list of people he had destroyed, and he was proud of his accomplishments. But David was confident he could overthrow his giant through the power of his God.

When you read the story in 1 Samual 17, notice how David encouraged himself by mentioning areas where he had achieved success. It is good to recognize your strengths before battle. David immediately proclaimed that he had killed a lion and a bear before. This was a new enemy, but it was the same concept.

The same faith in God you used to get a job, raise a child, or fight a bad reputation is the same weapon that is needed to overcome this enemy. You have what it takes, if you use it. The principles you used to overcome one thing can be used to overcome another. Giants are destroyed by those who refuse to be intimidated, know the power of God, and depend on Him to save them from destruction.

I know we are accustomed to using our faith against other problems, but today let's use faith to attack the thing that is attacking us. That means the first step to success with the body is our thinking. We build our faith to fight the giant in our own mind.

It is not important that we convince the giant we are going to win — it is important we convince ourselves. I know that I speak strong words about this foe, but for many people it is a formidable foe. We have conquered many other things, but this one thing snarls its teeth and glares at us every morning. We look at ourselves getting out of the shower or glimpse a side view in the mirror and we feel defeated.

Secret struggles are the worst because they are personal. When people address our secret grief, we resent their arrogance in taking liberties we have not granted. But we are not losing weight to prove anything to other people. This is done to prove to ourselves that we posses the stamina to endure and the tenacity to triumph. In so doing, we gain control of a part of our lives.

> Health is a state of complete physical, mental, and social well-being, and not merely the absence of disease or infirmity.
>
> Constitution, The World Health Organization

Lay aside the weight today — perhaps just to prove to yourself that you can. You will never be as young or as strong as you are today. Why not get started right now? Prepare your mind for battle. Better still, prepare your mind for winning! You are at this moment gathering the stones that will determine your success.

That giant, Goliath, was tall and strong, but he mistakenly appraised David's ability by looking at his demeanor. David wasn't threatening outwardly. Some-times we may not look like we have much strength if you judge us by the flesh. But David had a secret weapon. It was his faith in God.

Goliath never knew what hit him. It wasn't just the stones David threw, it was the faith with which he threw them. The stones were the truths he picked up along the way. They were natural, but they were thrown with supernatural force. We need to combine natural truths with supernatural truths.

In the following chapters, we will discuss the five smooth stones you can use to overcome the giant that is after you. They may be some things you have done before, but the stones alone are not the key. The stones combined with your faith become an unstoppable weapon. That giant won't know what hit him!

chapter 3

Call the Enemy's Bluff

Warfare against giants must be direct and bold!

Giants laugh at cowardice and weak attempts to thwart them. They defiantly proclaim their intent to take anything that brings us joy.

Perhaps the most intimidating aspect of giants is not their intent but their size. The giant is that huge issue in your life that seems insurmountable. It represents that "one thing" that parades around suggesting that it cannot be conquered.

Your giant is the issue that desires to dominate and control you and its stature is its first line of offense. The second is its threatening intention to devour you. But have no fear. If you are running from a giant, it is time to turn around and call his bluff.

It is easy to be intimidated by the enemy's appearance of power. Sometimes he may threaten to crush us with outside pressures in an attempt to steal our joy by making big victories seem insignificant and small in comparison to the task before us. He uses our susceptibility to stress and anxiety to make us feel helpless against him.

Many times it is not so much the giant's height or strength as much as it is our feelings of inferiority that make the giant seem so large. If some giant has you cornered, it is time to take back your right to the good life again. Isn't that really what freedom is all about? Taking back control of your life. We Christians need to be free to choose our direction without being controlled by our urges.

Those of us who have waged a war with our weight know the giant sometimes works through external pressures. Feelings of stress and anxiety find resolution in our taste buds rather than in our prayers and faith. The demands of our lives are pacified with the sedative offerings of sugars and food. Sometimes we eat without even being hungry. It is almost as if the giant demands we pay a toll for the stress through which he drives us.

As he pushes us to new boundaries and sizes, we start looking like giants ourselves! If you can leap in the air and feel yourself jiggling after your feet hit the ground, you know what I am saying. Whatever is left shaking when your feet hit the ground is the part that the giant is holding captive!

I ask myself the question, "Why even bother to discuss something so private and so personal as my battle with weight?" Whenever you write on an issue like this, people take liberties with you. They evaluate your success, comment on your size, and discuss your struggle as if they went to school with you.

I am basically a very private person. Why then would I want to discuss with

> Old age must be resisted, and its deficiencies supplied by taking pains; we must fight it as we do disease. Care must be bestowed upon health; moderate exercise should be taken; food and drink should be sufficient to recruit, not overburden, our strength. And not the body alone must be sustained, but the powers of the mind much more; unless you supply them, as oil to a lamp, they too grow dim with age. Whereas over-exertion weighs the body down with fatigue, exercise makes the mind buoyant.
>
> — Marcus Tullius Cicero

total strangers the details of my life? Why confess my own battles with one of the generational curses that desired to hold me prisoner and take my life? Why should I want to openly share these private parts of my life with people I do not know?

I normally would not think of doing it. But, as I briefly mentioned before, when I travel through airports and stay in hotels across the country, I see too many people who ask me how I lost the weight. Some are just encouraging me, but others are looking desperately to find a tool that will assist them in their plight with the giant that tries to dominate them. So I must push my personal preference for privacy to the side and reach out to others who need to gain a measure of control in their lives.

I have found five weapons to use against the enemy when he bullies me. For a little over ten years, he had convinced me that I could not lose weight, so I didn't even focus on it. I thought it was too difficult. I was too old. I was too busy. But that was a deception. The giant was bluffing me.

Once I got motivated to fight back, the first thing that amazed me was that the weight actually fell off. I admit I had to be motivated, but once I decided to fight, it was amazing how easily the weight lost its grip on my life and Goliath came tumbling down.

I want to pass these weapons on to you. To defeat this giant, we must first be mentally prepared for the fight against him. We need a reason to fight him and a purpose that is big enough to keep us from retreating. We need to focus on a clear mission to remind us why we want to be free from the giant when his threats begin to scare us.

Our motive for fighting the fat giant must be big enough to keep us from giving up. Being more physically attractive was not enough to motivate me. But when I realized he was trying to kill me, I thought, *Wait a minute! It is one thing to have to buy tents and cut them into suits. It is one thing to fly first class because your hind parts are jammed into coach seats. But it is another thing entirely to live your adult life hooked up to a dialysis machine over a piece of cheesecake!*

What Would You Rather Be Doing Right Now?

To establish a mission that is big enough to keep you in the fight for health and fitness, ask yourself, "What do I want to do or be more than anything else?" What are you after? If you have no goal you can have no success.

I do not mean a certain weight goal, though that is important. You need a goal relating to where you want to go in life and what you must do to get there. Ask yourself, "Why do I want to accomplish this goal?" This goal is what your giant wants to steal from you, and you will have to fight him to reach it.

Be sure you get your motivation to fight him from within *your own goal.* Other people wanting it for you does not work. Their concern turns to nagging, and trying to please them leads to sneaking food at three o'clock in the morning. My wife used to say that our kitchen counter looked like we had mice in the morning. Why? Because I had a tendency to get up in the middle of the night and help myself to just one more piece of that peach cobbler. Some people are sleepwalkers. I was an eat walker!

If you are reading this book because you want to lose weight, like I did, your answer to what you want most in your life may be that you want to become thin so you will look better. But what happens to that determination when loving people in your life reaffirm your attractiveness? I mean, there are people who will love you just as you are.

I am so blessed that I married someone who loves me unconditionally. Many of you may be surrounded by people who are just like that, or they may have similar struggles with weight. The overweight look can become a family earmark. Therefore, the stimulus cannot be predicated upon other peoples' view of you. This has to be *your* desire or forget it. It will not work.

> And whosoever of you will be the chiefest, shall be servant of all.
>
> For even the Son of Man came not to be ministered unto, but to minister, and to give his life a ransom for many.
>
> Mark 10:44,45

Perhaps you want to be thin in time for an upcoming holiday or a family reunion. But how many class reunions did you either decline or were reluctant to attend because you didn't reach your goal in time? Greater still, what will you do after the class reunion, but go back to the same lifestyle you had before? What happened to your determination to be thin when you attended the reunion and discovered that most of your friends had gained just as much as you had?

Wanting to lose weight so that you can buy a new dress or a smart looking suit is not a good reason to lose weight. The mission to be thin for the sake of appearance is easily thwarted by the giant, whose passion to destroy us is greater than our desire to be svelte.

If wanting to become thin is the only answer you can give me for desiring to lose weight at this time, let me ask you this question: What will you feel more like doing when you are thin that you don't feel like doing now?

Do you realize how much greater the quality of your life can be? I think the most surprising thing to me was how much younger I felt after losing nearly 100 pounds. I thought I was getting older. I was getting older, but weight adds years to your appearance and your performance. You just don't feel like doing anything for as long or as well as you would if you didn't have that bag of grits hanging off your hips!

The questions in this interrogation are worth meditating upon and thinking through until you reach a well-defined answer. Within the depths of exploring what you want to do with your life, you will find a motivating cause that is worth the sacrifice it may take to get to it. A little soul searching is good; it will take your inner strength to fight the giant.

When I first met my friend, health designer and chef Carlo Gabrelian, it wasn't because I wanted to lose weight. I just desired to help my wife with the demands of entertaining, raising five children, working everyday, and doing all of the other things that a pastor's wife over a large congregation has to contend with on a daily basis.

There simply weren't enough hours in the day for her to do all she used to do and still have time for Daddy. She thought Carlo was my gift to her. But freeing up a little of her time was as much a gift to me as it was to her. (Just don't tell her I had a selfish motive, okay?)

Carlo prepared whatever I requested, but he talked a lot about food choices. I learned so many things. I found out that knowledge is power. I gradually started thinking differently about food and its purpose. I think he was baiting me to take on the giant. Subtly, he just left me with the information I needed to gain the courage to attack what was attacking me. I had already lost 35 pounds on my own, so I was leaning in that direction. You do not have to have a trainer to lose weight, but I had lost all that I could lose with the knowledge I had.

I had hit a plateau and was gradually starting to think I could not lose any more weight without starving myself to death. To me that was not an option. To this day, I have been able to lose and keep off the weight without becoming hungry and spastic.

Carlo questioned why I wanted to lose weight, and he wanted a good reason. He explained, "Anyone can lose weight, and there are many ways to do it, but these wild faddish diets are simply an interruption to the lifestyle that led you to this state of poor health. As soon as you stop starving yourself and go back to your old lifestyle, it will bring everything back to the way it was. This back and forth gaining and losing ritual is bad for your heart. I don't believe in crash diets, but I will show you how to change your lifestyle."

Carlo taught me how to lay aside my weight by sharing amazing things that helped me understand my body and how it works and processes food. I then began to add what

I know about my faith and how to build up my spirit to take on challenges.

You see, everything you have to face must be challenged according to the power that works within you. It is a thrill to use my God-given graces for self-empowerment. Every pound was a victory as I began to use the knowledge of my body and the faith in my God to overthrow the enemy that was out to destroy the quality and the quantity of my life. I was getting control back, and man, was that a great feeling!

Giants are intensely personal — in your face. They tell you you will never succeed, that you will always be their slave.

Giants lie!

Again, the same faith you use in other areas of your life to attain victory is going to defeat this giant. You have God-given power within yourself to overcome. Most of you will not need the prescription drugs or the modern surgeries. You have faith in God — now let's exercise it! You have the power within you to overcome the enemy. That is why you need both the spiritual information that I am sharing, coupled with the physical information that Carlo provides to see the giant destroyed.

Carlo has trained Olympic team members in seventeen countries throughout the world. As he cooks for them, he also teaches them how to make wise choices on a daily basis so they will be finely tuned on the day of their big game. Food giants shake in their boots when they see his disciplined athletes come on to the playing field. His fitness disciples have ranged from boxers and rugby players to table tennis stars. Some wanted to be thin; some needed to be heavier. The outcome of their training depended on the game they wanted to win.

There is no right weight or look for you. If you are medically healthy, there is no perfect size appearance-wise that insures self-esteem. This is not an attempt to look like some designer's image of what they say is attractive. This is an exercise in restoring the decisions and control back to you. That is your body, God's temple, and as you seek Him, He will show you what changes are necessary for you to fulfill your purpose.

I know I didn't have time for the burden of weight. And I definitely didn't have time for the sicknesses that were circling like buzzards over my head, waiting to bring generational afflictions. I decided to take authority over the thing that was taking authority over me.

The mission that kept these Olympians from quitting was not the vanity gained from appearance, but the glory won from performance. Carlo can tell us many stories of athletes who took the decision of their health into their own control because they had learned the thrill of winning the game. But we need not hear their testimonies to believe God for our deliverance in this area of challenge. It is our faith in God that enables us to have the courage to pursue this and all other dreams in Jesus' name.

Receiving God's promise may be hindered by lack of discipline. Blessings often have boundaries of obedience. Your financial prosperity, relationships, and many other things God wants to do in your life may be affected by this one giant that is holding you hostage. I know there are some who have tremendous discipline and still see little results. But most of us know why we are not seeing the giant destroyed. The evidence can be seen in the crumbs left lying on the kitchen counter!

There are some people who struggle with food even though they are not being defeated through obesity. Sometimes the enemy steals the food away completely, and we suffer through anorexia or bulimia. Some people become listless because they haven't re-energized their body with efficient fuel that will take them where they want to go. They live in fear and have undue anxiety about weight gain. The enemy is destroying them with extremism.

Fear is not the motivation that is needed for weight control. When fear reigns, other disorders evolve. Do not be afraid to take on the enemy. Half of the battle depends on your faith. You cannot overcome him with fear, but with faith you can do anything.

Remember these scriptures that I share with you. Include them in your prayer time. Meditate on them as you prepare to destroy the giant. Here is a great scripture for you to hold onto as you prepare.

"And this is the victory that overcometh the world, even our faith."

1 John 5:4

Giants, those insurmountable challenges, have a clear mission. They want to steal and kill and destroy. But Jesus Christ came that we might have and enjoy life. It is written, in John 10:10, that Jesus meant for us to have life in abundance, to the point that it is overflowing. According to *Vine's Expository Dictionary of New Testament Words,* abundant life is described as the "God kind of life":

"LIFE, LIVING, LIFETIME, LIFE-GIVING"

1. ZOE (Eng., "zoo," "zoology") is used in the N.T. "of life as a principle, life in the absolute sense, life as God has it, that which the Father has in Himself, and which He gave to the Incarnate Son to have in Himself, John 5:26, and which the Son manifested in the world, 1 John 1:2. From this life man has become alienated in consequence of the Fall, Ephesians 4:18, and of this life men become partakers through faith in the Lord Jesus Christ, John 3:15, who becomes its Author to all such as trust in Him, Acts 3:15, and who is therefore said to be 'the life' of the believer, Colossians 3:4, for the life that He gives He maintains, John 6:35, 63."

Christ came to restore that which was lost in the fall. Every area of our lives that we yield to Him becomes another place for us to experience life as God intended it for us. The resurrection power of God is there to assist us in recovering what the enemy has stolen. God's power is like dynamite ready to explode the traps that were set by Satan to snare you.

> I am come that they might have life, and that they might have it more abundantly.
>
> John 10:10

When was the last time you felt like you had too much energy? When is the last time you woke up with an eagerness to bounce out of bed because you felt too good to lie there any longer? If you can't remember, then watch out, there may be a giant staking out your dream. He intends to take it from you unless you destroy him first.

You can destroy your enemy just like David destroyed Goliath. All you need is a slingshot, which is the power of your faith; a good aim at your real enemy, which is discernment; and a few solid river stones to weaken and ultimately destroy your giant, which are truths from God's Word.

In this book, I explain the truths that empowered me to change. They are very simple. As Carlo explained the concepts of managing my weight, which included mental preparation, restrictive intake, adaptation, maintenance, and balance, I could see biblical lessons that would also help my brothers and sisters in Christ experience health and well-being.

I call these spiritual truths the five smooth stones I used to slay the giant that was trying to stop my ministry and steal my joy of life. I now carry these stones with me to defeat any giant that rises up against me. Together these stones of truth defeated my obesity, so I continue to use them against other obstacles that hinder my ability to receive God's best for my life.

I am going to put these five smooth stones in your bag. Then the Holy Spirit is going to use them to help you slay this and any other giant that would come against you.

chapter 4

Collect your Weapons!

An accurate aim shortens the war.

Having the right reason for losing weight advances your success in winning the prize you are after. You must determine exactly what it is you want so that when the enemy laughs in your face, you won't forget your reason for standing firmly against him. Motivation is the first stone you need to pick up for your battle.

Let me ask you the question again: If you were already fit and healthy, what would you be doing that you aren't doing right now? What would you do if you felt good enough to do it? Would you take your children to the park more often? Would you say yes when they ask you to join in a game of volleyball in the front yard?

Would you keep a tidier house? Would you exude more confidence in your relationship with your spouse? How do you think weight control would help strengthen your relationships?

Would you apply for the promotion you have been wanting at the office? More accurately, would you be more apt to be hired for that position if your appearance were different? I know it seems unfair that appearance is a factor in hiring, but it is. They will never admit it, but it is a factor.

There is a certain image that most secular companies want to exemplify. Many times their reluctance is that they immediately assume overweight people are going to be a health risk and prone to be sick. Of course we know that this is an unfair assumption. Yet it does happen.

If you felt better, would you be more likely to volunteer when the vacation Bible school director was begging for helpers? Sitting on the floor playing games with your children and running behind them while they ride bicycles in the park is easier when you feel better. Would you feel more like being a sponsor for the youth retreat next fall?

When shopping, would you try a particular style of dress or shorts or jeans you now avoid because your weight prohibits you from feeling comfortable in them? Would you pack your bags and take that vacation to the islands? Perhaps you would even stand up before the congregation and tell your testimony more often — that is, if you only felt better about yourself. The enemy wants to keep you from enjoying this quality of life.

Decide What Game You Want to Win

Carlo told me that the first phase of training for my new lifestyle was psychological preparation. He said I needed to know why I wanted to make a change. I needed to find a motivation that was big enough and strong enough to defeat the tempter when he tried to take away my mission. He asked me, "What game do you want to win?" I might not ever train for the Olympics, but this was my challenge, nonetheless, to take on this marathon.

It made sense scripturally. The Bible says we are transformed by the renewing of our minds. (See Romans 12:2.) I wanted to be transformed because my body had been conformed to a size 56 suit. That is a lot of "conformed."

Now I needed to transform my body by the renewing of my mind, because it all starts with a decision. It starts with a motivated choice. I decided with my mind, then dominated my body until it was transformed to what I had in my mind. Notice this concept in the Word. It focuses around presenting your body as a living sacrifice.

"I beseech you therefore, brethren, by the mercies of God, that ye present your bodies a living sacrifice, holy, acceptable unto God, which is your reasonable service.

"And be not conformed to this world: but be ye transformed by the renewing of your mind, that ye may prove what is that good, and acceptable, and perfect, will of God."

Romans 12:1,2

It was a sacrifice that I needed to present to God. God is more glorified by living sacrifices than by shortened lives. I wanted Him to use me, but I needed to make certain changes in order to have the stamina to serve Him. It wasn't for image that it needed to be done, but for my health and ministry. For me, that was a great motivation. And besides, who doesn't want to look their best?

No matter what the challenge is in life, you cannot meet it without being motivated to succeed. When God was preparing Israel to conquer the Promised Land, He required them to send spies over to view what they were

> ... head hunger (this urge to eat when the body is not calling for it) is not true physiological hunger, but rather is spiritual hunger. So we learn how to replace it with the Word of God so that you transfer this urge for a pan of brownies to that of hungering and thirsting after righteousness.
>
> — Gwen Shamblin, M.S., R.D., Founder of The Weigh Down Workshop

Collect your Weapons!

going to conquer. He knew that a motivated people are a conquering people. He knew that whenever we are motivated to succeed, we are relentless to conquer. So He wanted them to taste the grapes from where they were going. This text is one of the greatest motivational stories I have ever read.

"And they returned from searching of the land after forty days.

"And they went and came to Moses, and to Aaron, and to all the congregation of the children of Israel, unto the wilderness of Paran, to Kadesh; and brought back word unto them, and unto all the congregation, and shewed them the fruit of the land.

"And they told him, and said, We came unto the land whither thou sentest us, and surely it floweth with milk and honey; and this is the fruit of it.

"Nevertheless the people be strong that dwell in the land, and the cities are walled, and very great: and moreover we saw the children of Anak there.

"The Amalekites dwell in the land of the south: and the Hittites, and the Jebusites, and the Amorites, dwell in the mountains: and the Canaanites dwell by the sea, and by the coast of Jordan.

"And Caleb stilled the people before Moses, and said, Let us go up at once, and possess it; for we are well able to overcome it."

Numbers 13:25-30

Don't be afraid to see yourself at the size and in the shape you want to be. Get a clear picture of your dream in your mind. Make plans for it. This battle will not be won at the table or in the gym. It will be won in your mind. It is won when you set your face toward the Promised Land and decide you are going to drive that giant back out of your house.

The battle is won by holding up your promise of abundant life and saying, "I want it. I want it now! I don't want to get ill to lose weight. I do not want to staple my stomach or mutilate myself through strange drugs. I want it by faith. The just shall live by faith. I will have it by faith. Amen."

An Acronym for Staying M-O-T-I-V-A-T-E-D!

M — is for mornings. Morning is the most crucial time to fight life's giants, because it is what you do in the morning that will influence the remainder of your day. I used to think I was too busy to eat breakfast, but breakfast is a significant meal. It helps to regulate you so you will eat at the proper times throughout the day. Most people who do not eat breakfast eat more and more later in the day. The evening is their ravenous time.

Reroute your appetite by taking advantage of your heightened metabolism in the morning. Enjoy a hearty but healthy breakfast. Though breakfast is a great time to fuel up, most breakfast foods are loaded with fat. Check the recipes in the back of this book for healthy alternatives, but please do not miss the mornings. You need a healthy hearty breakfast every morning.

O — is for the organization of your refrigerator. You must get rid of the Fat Team. They are the mayonnaise-based sauces, butters, cheeses, and oils that are in there to entice you. They can be replaced with fat-free equivalents. Many fat-free dressings taste so good, you will not notice a significant difference. These products will enable your family to continue eating the style of food they are accustomed to without giving the giant a hand.

> Keep healthy foods like fruit and vegetables handy. Set a schedule for meals and snacks that is right for you.

Most of your fat grams are coming from things you could replace and not miss! In order to do this you have to go to the grocery store on a mission to reorganize your shelves for the fight. After all, who would go to war without organizing their weapons. C'mon, get out of that house and arm yourself for the fight!

T — is for the time you must invest in your own health. It is not going to be a lot of time, but it will be beneficial. There are 168 hours in a week. You only need to exercise a total of 4 hours each week, one hour every other day. It is better to invest one whole hour at a pace that gets your heart rate up and keeps it up for one hour, than to break it into 30-minute or 15-minute intervals.

Short workouts may be more convenient, but they are far less effective. Carlo says that it takes approximately 30 minutes of exercise before you start burning into the stored fat in your body. Only after that amount of time will you decrease your size. It doesn't have to be painful exercise, just a consistent exercise at a good steady pace. I increased my pace with time.

I found the hard part was not the effort but the boredom. I kept thinking that I could be doing other things. I learned to enhance it by adding something I enjoy to what I honestly just endured. I tried watching action movies while I walked the treadmill. It made it easier for me by distracting me from the monotony of the routine.

I — is for the **information** with which you need to surround yourself. Remember, this battle is fought in the mind as much as the body. Arm your mind with knowledge such as we are sharing in this book.

The more I understood about my body and how it processes food, the better I could fight the giant. I was ignorant of the enemy's devices. I didn't know how my own body was processing food. To not know the truth is to fight in the dark. No wonder we lose. We either do not know, or we learn everything from the people who are only trying to sell us their food.

V — is for the **vision** you need to keep in front of you as a reminder of where you are going. No one can drive with the windows fogged up. Vision determines your direction. A strong vision of what you are going to be doing, what you will look like, and how you are going to feel will help you combat the other vision that tries to ensnare you.

You know the giant's vision, the one of the strawberries running down the sides of the three-inch-high piece of cheesecake. It is the vision that tries to lure us from our dream by tempting us with southern fried chicken with its golden brown crispy crust, served with the creamy potatoes smothered in gravy made from the fatty grease in which the chicken was fried.

Collect your Weapons!

You need a vision to counteract the giant's vision that wants to drag you back! No wonder the Bible says that without a vision the people perish. (See Proverbs 29:18.) I don't know about perishing, but I do know that if you do not keep the *right* vision in front of you, you will be sitting on mounds of fat behind you!

A — is for the places and people you must avoid. There are some people who see your dietary change as a challenge. They will want to set you up to fall. They do not mean any harm; they just get a kick out of seeing you cheat. I learned to eat before I went out to dinner so that I would not be at the mercy of the host. I learned to avoid putting myself in situations where I would be apt to fall.

This might not be a good time to go visit Grandma's house, especially since she keeps a can of grease on the stove to add to her vegetables. You know how she likes to make macaroni and cheese with so much butter, the pasta needs a bathing suit to swim in all the fat grams. Invite her to *your* house.

Avoid situations, restaurants, and people who present high temptations for you — at least until you have seen enough results to look them in the face and say, "No. Your offer is not worth my losing what I have seen God do in my life."

T — is for the temperance you have to use in learning to stop eating before your stomach inflates and your body wants to go to bed. We have often conditioned ourselves to eat more than we need, into the oblivion of indulgence. We have to learn to be temperate. It takes about twenty minutes for your brain to get the message that your stomach is satisfied. You would be surprised how much damage you can do at a table in twenty minutes. So practice being temperate.

E — is for seizing extra opportunities to strengthen your energy and burn off extra calories. It includes taking the stairs over the elevator. It includes parking further from the door and allowing yourself to walk. It includes picking up the pace just a bit when you walk and never driving the car when your destination is within a mile of you.

D — is for the determination you have to accomplish the goal, vanquish the foe, and deliver the praise back to the God Who helped you to do it. You are determined, aren't you? Then go for it!

There is no limitation on the life of someone who will not quit. It is that determination that caused David to destroy Goliath. It is that determination that allowed Joshua to get to the land that flowed with milk and honey (I am sure it was 2 percent milk)! Whatever it takes, go for it. You will have more self-respect when you keep your word to yourself!

I had good reason to fight the giant. I had a lot of motivation. I wanted to avoid the sickbed where I saw my father waste away before he finally died. Abundant life became my motivation for staying in the battle against the giant that growled within me, asking for more food.

> Motivation was enough for David to enter the battle, but his understanding was the power to win it.

I wanted the abundant life more than I wanted beans and corn bread! I wanted abundant life more than I wanted late night fellowship dinners after church. Eventually, I learned to fellowship without paying the price of French silk chocolate pie. I wanted to live a long and healthy life more than I wanted the sweet, but brief, taste of indulgence. Don't let me keep you from enjoying your dessert — it doesn't even tempt me in light of the game I am going to win.

What Is Your Motivation?

Finding the right motivation is the first step of psychological preparation for any battle. Saul tried to find ways to motivate his men to fight Goliath. He declared, "I'll make you wealthy if you kill Goliath. Yeah, and you can marry my daughter. And I won't even charge you taxes on the deal!" (See 1 Samuel 17:25.) But no man wanted any of Saul's rewards badly enough to fight the giant. They were terrified and dismayed by the giant's words.

When David heard Goliath chant his usual threats, David asked, "What shall be done to the man that killeth this Philistine, and taketh away the reproach from Israel? for who is this uncircumcised Philistine, that he should defy the armies of the living God?" (1 Samuel 17:26).

As soon as David proclaimed his interest in killing the giant, his own brother, Eliab, rose up against him, challenging his motives. In verse 28, he accused David of being conceited and irresponsible. "You're supposed to be watching the sheep. You aren't even supposed to be here. Who do you think you are anyway?" Doesn't that sound like the accuser who attacks our resolutions to change the unfavorable circumstances in our lives?

David's father was worried about his sons who were at war, so David came to check on their welfare. Before leaving the sheep at home, he put them in good care of another shepherd. His reason for being on the battlefield was to take food from their father's table to his brothers. (See 1 Samuel 17:17,18.)

David wasn't afraid of the giant, as his next response revealed, "Let no man's heart fail because of him; thy servant will go and fight with this Philistine" (1 Samuel 17:32). David was the youngest, but his actions showed maturity and responsibility towards others.

What Was David's Motivation?

David loved God with all his heart, and he loved others more than his own life. I guess you could say that David loved God and his fellowmen more than he loved his mother's home-cooked meals. He didn't say, "I would fight you, Goliath, but I have to be home in time for dinner." No, David wasn't afraid of missing a meal, but he did fear the name of the Lord — and he didn't want God's people to fall into bondage again.

David's motive was love, and love casts out fear. (1 John 4:19.) You need a motivation that is bigger than your fear of the giant, so choose love. Find someone or some dream to love more than life, and let it motivate your mission to become a person whose life is a testimony to what God can do with those who trust Him.

I love my family more than I love satisfying my appetite for old foods that were detrimental to my health. I want to be around to see my loved ones enjoying God's blessing. The food I was eating was robbing me of my health and energy. The bigger I grew, the more fearful I became that I might miss out on what God had laid up for me here on earth. But I'm not afraid of giants anymore.

Who Do You Love More than Life?

Many times we think that what we do in the privacy of our own time is our own business. That may be true, but our decisions will always have an effect on someone else. As I look back to the time I had to watch my dad die, I can see that the decision he made to neglect his high blood pressure had a terrifying impact on our family.

> Measure your health by your sympathy with morning and spring. If there is no response in you to the awakening of nature — if the prospect of an early morning walk does not banish sleep, if the warble of the first bluebird does not thrill you — know that the morning and spring of your life are past. Thus may you feel your pulse.
>
> Henry David Thoreau

Take this stone of motivation as your first weapon against the thief who wants to take your life. A bag of stones may not look intimidating to a giant — even Goliath laughed at David — but a small stone in the hand of someone who believed God won freedom for an entire nation. Though David was only a young boy at the time, his motivation to slay the giant was stronger than any temptation to run at the last minute.

Goliath had made a deal with Israel. Look at the story in 1 Samuel 17:9. The giant's wager read something like this: "If you kill me, then all my people will serve you. If you lose, you and your people will serve us." Doesn't that sound like Satan? "If I win, you serve me; if you win, I serve you!"

David's motivation was clear: If he won, he kept his freedom; if he lost, he became a slave. How hard would you fight if the stakes were that high? David knew the battle wasn't about making him look good in the eyes of those who watched. He fought to keep his entire nation free from bondage to the Philistines.

Carlo has had many clients come to him for help, but he was especially pleased by one mother. She quickly discovered her true motivation for wanting to be fit after only spending a few hours with him. Her hope had been dimmed from the many diets she had tried over the past fifteen years, only to fail again and again. By the time she met Carlo, her regrets had increased, because now her failure was being passed on to her children.

She had three beautiful children who had suffered the consequences of too many pizza deliveries and trips to fast food drive-ins as a result of their busy life. They all lacked energy, were short-tempered, and fought embarrassment for being heavier than their peers at school.

Condemnation on the mother was mounting, because now her lifestyle affected more than her personal health. Her poor eating habits brought shame on her children who had to eat the food she set before them. She finally realized her victory over poor eating habits would win the game of life for her children and husband too.

After only a few weeks of using these five stones, she reported that her entire family was enjoying better meals, fewer fights between the siblings, and trimmer waistlines.

Satan hasn't changed. He still challenges you to serve him or defeat him. It doesn't matter what the battle is. You could be fighting your weight, an impulse to spend money you don't have, or time-wasters that keep you from investing in steps that lead to a more fulfilling life.

Use the right motivation of love to encourage yourself to face the giant. Killing giants saves more lives than just your own! Go ahead, throw this first stone of motivation at the devil. Catch him by surprise and refuse him the next time he tempts you.

Rejoice and celebrate even the smallest victories over him. I still pat myself on the back when I choose blackened salmon and fat-free dressing over a 16-ounce steak with a fully loaded baked potato.

Remind the devil that it is written: Man shall not live by bread alone, but by every word that proceeds from the mouth of God. (See Matthew 4:4.)

Take a moment right now to find your highest motivation for slaying the giant that has stolen your self-control.

What do you want more than being a slave to your appetite?

Who are the people in your life who are waiting for you to feel better?

Describe a perfect day and keep the vision of it before you.

Who do you know who would love to go for a walk with you?

Take a walk sometime today and write down how it made you feel.

chapter 5

Grip Your Slingshot!
Weapons needed for giant-slaying are simple.

David defeated Goliath with a slingshot and five water-polished stones. He refused the armor Saul gave to him and didn't seem too impressed with the rewards the king offered to the one who killed the giant. Goliath had bellowed his challenge for forty days, but no man wanted to marry a princess badly enough to fight this ten-foot mass of ruthless flesh.

Look again at the story in 1 Samuel 17. David came to see his brothers and heard everyone talking about the giant. The king's men said, "Have you seen this man who has come out to defy Israel? To the man who kills this giant, the king will give great riches, his daughter's hand in marriage, and make his father's house free from taxes and service in Israel!"

David spoke to the men and said, "But what shall be done for the man who kills this Philistine and removes this disgrace from Israel?"

And the men repeated the recompense again, perhaps thinking, *What part of riches, fame, and the easy-life from here on out do you not understand, brother?* Maybe David just didn't hear them the first time, or maybe he was saying, "All those promises could be won without killing giants. So, what is the real reward?" Either way, David understood something the other men didn't.

- David understood that killing the giant was part of a much bigger purpose and plan of God than the gratuity the king could offer.
- David understood that killing this giant won freedom for all of Israel and glorified God.
- David understood that Goliath wasn't anymore powerful than the lion and bear he had fought in earlier battles.
- David understood that it was the Lord Who had delivered him out of the paw of the lion and out of the paw of the bear.
- David understood that the Lord would deliver him out of the hand of the Philistine.

> No matter what field we choose for our careers or what our mission is in life, we need to have physical conditioning to see it through.
>
> — A. C. Green

When he marched onto the field, David took his faithful slingshot, the one he had used in earlier battles. He chose river stones he knew would be accurate, top-flight performers when hurled through the air. And he trusted God to be his only shield. He had faith in his hand, truth in his pocket, and God's impenetrable protection encompassed about him. David's understanding set him apart from all the king's men.

"Understanding" Is the Second Stone

Imagine Goliath's surprise when, after forty days of boasting and challenging Saul's men to a play-off, he sees a young unarmored boy walk on the field with what appeared to be a stick.

Goliath said the same thing to David that we have heard the devil say to us, "Come to me, and I will give your flesh to the birds of the air and the beasts of the field."

Then David replied, "You come to me with powerful looking weapons, but I come to you in the name of the Lord of hosts, the God of Israel, Whom you have defied. Today, the Lord will deliver you into my hand."

- David understood Who God was and what His will was for His people.
- David understood that God did not want His people to be slaves to the Philistines.
- David understood God's bigger plan.
- David understood that truth was the jab that would weaken his opponent.
- David understood that God's glory was being challenged.
- David understood that God would defend His own name.

How Clear Is Your Understanding of This Battle of the Bulge?

"Wisdom is the principal thing; therefore get wisdom: and with all thy getting get understanding.

"Exalt her, and she shall promote thee: she shall bring thee to honour, when thou dost embrace her.

"She shall give to thine head an ornament of grace: a crown of glory shall she deliver to thee."

Proverbs 4:7-9

Our war on weight is much the same. Our weapons can be as simple as having a right motivation and an understanding of how food affects the way we feel about the things we want to do in life. When I understood that the person I wanted to be and things I wanted to do had a direct relationship with the food I chose to nourish my body, I began to view food differently.

One of the things that helped me to get an understanding was the effect of my culture on my eating habits. African Americans, like many other cultures in our society, celebrate most major events with food. We bring food when babies are born; we bring food when people die. We celebrate every holiday with food, and most of our family outings and events are surrounded by lots of fat-filled, sugar-loaded, festive-type foods.

I began to realize that I associated good times with eating. My first challenge, therefore, was to develop good times that were not inundated with fatty foods. I had to realize that in some cases, it is possible to celebrate without food. I believe we have all been conditioned to associate food with good feelings. The problem with that is food was given for nourishment. There needs to be a clear line of distinction between feelings and food. I wasn't eating to supply my body with energy. I was eating because I associated food with fun.

Beyond the cultural influences I was raised to enjoy, I additionally had to fight the influences of the Christian church. Most Christians develop life styles that are built around worship services and late night fellowships. These fellowships require you to eat large meals after 10 p.m. Again, the atmosphere is festive, and the presence of food seems to be a mandate for each occasion. I needed to understand the difference between fun and fuel.

When I was 338 pounds, I was at the height of my ministry. We were conducting crusades and keeping up with extensive television schedules. My burden of weight didn't stop me from ministering, but it certainly kept me from enjoying it. I felt good about what God was doing. I felt good about the spiritual man he was raising up inside of me. But I wavered between not feeling good about my appearance and just plain not feeling physically fit.

It was not so much that I lacked energy. It was that once I was tired, I did not re-energize as quickly as I thought I should. For a man my size, I had always had an inordinate amount of energy. But once that was depleted, I noticed that my recuperating time was a lot more extensive than it had been. Now, after shedding so much excess weight, my recuperating time is much less.

I will never forget walking through the airport in Charlotte and reading a sign that so graphically depicted the realism of my life. It said, "Busy people don't have time for the weight." It was then that I suddenly began to understand I was too busy to be carrying all of these pockets, layers, suitcases, and potato sacks around my waist, hips, lips and finger tips. As captain of this

"He who gets wisdom loves his own soul; he who cherishes understanding prospers."
Proverbs 19:8 NIV

sinking ship, I decided to throw the bags off the sides and sail forward towards my destiny.

"The body is like a machine," Carlo said to me. "It is a very smart machine that takes the food that it is given and turns it into energy. It is simple mathematics. If the body gets more calories and fat than it can use, it has to put that food somewhere, faithfully believing that you want to store it away for some future famine. Then you will call for the extra energy to be used." My problem was that the future famine never came, and the fat account kept drawing interest until I could see the "growing" dividends bursting over my belt.

In other words, my body was saving the fat for a rainy day that never came. It stored all the excess it could not use into fat cells. When all the fat cells were full, the body created new fat cells. As I began to understand this, I was better prepared to liquidate the fat accounts and lay aside the weight. If I had known twenty years ago what I know now, this overwhelming fat pool may never have formed.

Regretfully, however, it had already happened. But now I was learning something I didn't understand before. Carlo has a passion for making people understand why it is important to eat right. He explained that a double hamburger with cheese contained 63 grams of fat. When I add mayonnaise, it's another 23 grams of fat! Throw in fries and a milkshake with another 27 grams, and I've just eaten 113 grams of fat in one meal!

After learning that, I didn't even want to tell Carlo what I had eaten for breakfast! I knew hamburgers and French fries were bad for me, but I didn't understand why until I took an honest look at what I was eating.

Because of my busy schedule, I had developed the habit of stopping at the drive-thru windows of fast food restaurants, snatching a greasy bag full of fat grams and devouring the stuff with one hand, while driving to the next appointment with the other.

Our ignorance of the truth can be devastating to our waistline and our energy. I just didn't understand what I was eating and what it was doing to my body. But when I did, I suddenly knew why my body had to work so hard to digest a meal and put all that extra fat somewhere for later use. I could see the little fat cells talking to each other saying, "Put a label on this case for the year 2025. It will be a good vintage by then!" Imagine the amount of fat grams we may be eating in one day without being aware of it.

Carlo teaches his clients to start reading the labels on the foods they love to eat. It is amazing how quickly the fat grams tally. On the contrary, a great deal of food can be eaten before the calorie limit is reached. I now understand there are many foods which are low in fat, high in flavor, and easy for my overworked body to digest. As I began to eat better food, my body began to rejuvenate and become strong again.

Now I make better choices because I understand why some foods help me achieve the tasks I am determined to do. I also understand that the enemy would like to throw my flesh to the birds of the air. But I choose to stay alive and fight for the kingdom of God. My body no longer has to work so hard to turn food into storage buckets of fat.

I understand that if I eat too much, I owe my body the service of finding ways to help use up those calories without refilling the fat cells. I do this by cutting back on my next meals and exercising.

Are You Tired of Being Tired?

The next two chapters will explain more specifically how to attack your weight problem and learn to make healthy choices. As you read them, you will pick up two more stones to use as an arsenal in your actual weight loss — conviction and knowledge.

Most health guides recommend that highly active people of normal weight who want to keep from gaining more should limit their calories to 2,400 calories a day with no more than 25% of their total calories in fat. This would be about 67 grams of fat per day. If a person wants to lose weight gradually, the nutrionists recommend that women eat between 20 and 40 grams of fat a day, and men 30 to 60 grams.

For now, remember to talk to your doctor first and let him know you are ready to lay aside the weight. He will help you set the right daily caloric intake and per-cent of fat grams that is right for your size and special needs.

You will find that the knowledge we share in how to lose weight is not so unusual. We'll discuss the common sense approach to gradual loss and counting calories and fat grams. What Carlo's methods did for me that other diets didn't was they opened my eyes to understand the truth of balance, moderation, and the benefit of low-fat foods in my diet.

We want to be sure your motivation is clear, that you understand this is a new lifestyle and not just a diet that interrupts the destructive path you may now be taking.

When I listed the goals that motivated me the most, I could see why my body was too tired to march to new horizons. I had made it work so hard just to digest my lunch!

A Lie Is A Heavy Weight to Carry

Our ignorance of the truth can be devastating to our waistline and our level of energy. But understanding can pull down barriers that keep us from moving on.

What misconceptions about food are weighing you down? Whatever reason caused you to be overweight, you must first understand that obesity is a dangerous circumstance that leads to heart disease, strokes, and some forms of cancer. This is not part of God's design for us.

Some of us have believed a lie about food. We have justified our belt size with explanations like, "It doesn't matter what I eat. I still get fat from it. I think it's something to do with my family's genetics."

But God said food was good. Through a vision He gave to Peter, He even lifted the list of restrictive foods He had previously told the Israelites to avoid. (See Acts 10:9-16.) So family's tendency to be overweight is more likely to be from the family recipes than from a design of God.

We must also understand that everything from generational curses to badly formed habits is broken with the name of Jesus, just as David broke the giant's curse against Israel in the name of the Lord.

Maybe you're a victim of office parties, church potlucks, and a group of friends who love to go out to eat together. It is true that we all eat one half as much when we are alone than when we are with a group of people. However, food is not the only reward of fellowship. So choose from the light menu, take fat-free dressings to the office, and stay away from eating a sample of every dessert at the church spread.

Understanding Sees the Truth

The lure of food does not have the power over me now that it used to. I can look at a piece of cake and discern if it can help or hinder me in the task I want to do. I now understand that I can be a person who eats well or poorly, and the choices I make determine the person I will become.

If you view fat-laden foods as a hindrance, you can look at cake as an inedible object that holds no power of temptation over you. When you understand that vitamin rich fruits and vegetables will build your energy so you will enjoy your family more, you can see that the right food becomes inviting and pleasing to the eye.

Remember, you are not the enemy. You're a victim of a tempter who has been around for a long time. Food was the first thing the devil used to tempt Eve. Adam didn't hold up against the temptation when Eve said, "Look at what we can have if we eat this food." And eating something they knew they shouldn't had fatal consequences.

Eating the food God had made for them would have kept Adam and Eve where they wanted to be. But their lack of self-control lost everything that was worth having. The devil promised them that his food would take them where they wanted to go, but he is a deceitful thief.

Now for those of you who have been mad at Adam and Eve for losing our place in paradise, let me ask you, "Could you have resisted the devil if you were the one fighting for the freedom of mankind?" No, we've already proven that we wouldn't have lasted long in Eden. But God, in His great mercy and grace, knew we needed help, so He sent Jesus.

Food was the first temptation the devil tried against Jesus, but Jesus refused to satisfy his hunger from his forty-day fast with the devil's food. The devil used food to challenge Jesus to prove Who He was — the Son of God. Look at Matthew 4:3.

> "And when the tempter came to him, he said, If thou be the Son of God, command that these stones be made bread.
>
> But he answered and said, It is written, Man shall not live by bread alone, but by every word that proceedeth out of the mouth of God."
>
> Matthew 4:3,4

Jesus understood there was a bigger meal planned at His Father's table that was worth waiting for. He knew the devil's dessert would spoil the taste of His approaching wedding feast.

Did you know that a taco salad with sour cream can contain 59 grams of fat?

Jesus knew He didn't want to eat stones when His Father's table would offer a feast big enough for the whole Church to attend. I hope you will understand this same truth in winning the battle over self-indulgence. The devil would like for us all to eat the stones we are using against him. But don't forget that stones aren't for eating; they are for throwing at giants who want to steal our rightful inheritance.

Don't spoil your appetite by eating stones when you could have the bread of life! Discern the difference between the food that helps and food that hinders your path to the Wedding Feast of the Lamb.

"Then said they unto him, Lord, evermore give us this bread."

John 6:34

God's Burden is Light!

One of Carlo's clients called to tell him how great he felt after losing his first sixteen pounds, even though he had forty pounds to go. With excitement he explained, "Carlo, my briefcase weighs eight pounds. The weight I lost is like setting down a briefcase from each shoulder." And to think, I used to carry the equivalent of twelve of those cases on my own body day after day, night after night. God never intended for me to be so heavily yoked. Jesus said:

"Come unto me, all ye that labour and are heavy laden, and I will give you rest.

"Take my yoke upon you, and learn of me; for I am meek and lowly in heart: and ye shall find rest unto your souls.

"For my yoke is easy, and my burden is light."

Matthew 11:28-30

How many briefcases have you been carrying into battle? Isn't it time to trade yokes with Jesus?

As I cross the bridge to gaining control over my eating habits, I do it consciously aware of the fact that this is an ongoing process. Unlike some people, who seem to be able to eat whatever they want and not gain weight, I will, for whatever reason, remain a person who has an ongoing challenge to control the thing that desires my control.

I certainly don't want to brag, because the war isn't over. But I do think it would be nice to pause in the battle with self-indulgence long enough to encourage others. If we trust in God and follow His Word, we can overcome personal challenges just as we overcome moral failures.

I want to close this chapter with a word of prayer, asking God to give you the grace to face each day renewed in your mind by the Word of God, which promises that we can do all things through Christ Who strengthens us.

Father, I thank You for my brothers and sisters who, like me, have faced the giant. I thank You, Lord, that giants are never giants to You. As we look at them through Your eyes, the giants shrink before us. I pray that each person who reads this book will look at their giant through Your eyes and sling the stones of faith at the enemy in Your name.

Lord, I thank You that You have used my ministry to loose many people from many pains. Use this word today to loose those who struggle with their own flesh as it relates to obesity and any other temptation that might hinder them from maximizing every day You have given them. In the name of the Lord, Jesus, we pray. Amen.

chapter 6

Leave the Extra Luggage Behind!

Confidence consumes cowardice
when you are convinced of victory.

Courage is only needed if you aren't sure of yourself. If you doubt you can resist tempting foods when you begin the fight for your health, your battle will be unnecessarily difficult. Doubt is heavy baggage to carry into war, so you need to be *convinced* that self-control wins immeasurable rewards.

Once you understand that what you eat will either help or hinder your success in winning the freedom to enjoy the best of life, you won't need to depend on willpower to resist the foods that aren't healthy for you. Conviction will keep you on the winning side of the battleground.

- David was convinced God would support his acts of faith.
- David was convinced of the truth when he confronted Goliath.
- David was convinced that his slingshot was sufficient, because he had conquered other foes with this simple weapon of defense.

- David was convinced that smooth stones washed in water were better weapons than dirty ragged rocks.

Likewise, we know that knowledge washed with the water of God's Word (the Truth) is better than facts dug up from worldly experience. David was convinced that by acting on what he knew to be true, he would be set free from the threat of the enemy. And the same is true for us. Our part is to *believe* — God's part is to *do*.

Conviction Is the Third Stone

You must have a conviction that this time you take on the "Fat Master," you are going to succeed. The enemy will try to weaken your constitution by reminding you of past failures. The Lord knows the devil is a master at bringing up your past! But you must have a conviction that this is not like those other times.

Why? Because this time you are going to fight with the weapons the Lord gave you. This is not a battle that is to be fought through some secular-devised program that people who do not believe in prayer run toward. This is not a battle to be won through pills and drugs.

> All you have to do to lose weight is mix plenty of self-control with everything you eat.
>
> — Anonymous

This is a battle that is going to be won by faith in God's Word while maintaining a conviction that His principles for your life work. I know your weapons might seem meager, but just because they look *meager* doesn't mean they are not *mighty!*

What we believe in and are convicted of has power over us, whether it is the truth or a lie. Some may argue, "But doesn't truth rule over us whether we believe it or not?

Doesn't truth always win?" Let me tell you a parable that illustrates the power of believing the truth or a lie.

There was a man who lived on an island that had only one grocer who imported food for everyone who lived there. The man had no way to leave the island to purchase additional food and was totally dependent on the provision of the store in order to survive.

Then one day an evil, rumor-bearing neighbor told him the shelves of the grocer were bare, and because of famine on the mainland, there would be no more shipments of food. Instead of walking the few miles to the store himself, the man believed the report and simply laid down on his bed and waited for death to come.

The man was weak and near to death when a kind islander passed his hut on the way to the island's grocer. Glancing through the open door, he saw the very thin man lying on his bed in the middle of a bright and beautiful day.

Seeing the man's condition, he called to him, "Why are you lying there? Why are you starving here alone?"

The man explained that because there was no food on the island, he had decided to die quickly in the comfort of his own hut.

"But there is plenty of food to eat. There is no famine, and the ship comes every week as it has always done," the good neighbor explained. "There is plenty of nourishing food for you. Look at me and you will see that I am strong, well-fed, and nourished by the abundance of food I have received from the store. Your food is within an hour's walk from here."

But the man had been blinded by his starvation and could not see the truth. In his last breath he scorned the kind neighbor and demanded that he be left alone, "You only torment me with the hope of food that is not there. Leave me now and let me die."

Why did the man starve to death?

Was it because of the lie, or was it his conviction about an untruth?

Why didn't truth have the power to save him?

What Is Destroying Your Health?

If we believe it doesn't matter what we eat, our belief allows us to eat the wrong food. But if we are convinced that eating fatty-foods is dangerous to our health, we are empowered to resist the foods that bring us harm, and we willingly choose the foods that bring us health and abundant energy.

A lie has no power over us — unless we believe it. Unfortunately, truth has the same restrictions. Jesus said that we would *know* the truth and it would set us free. (See John 8:32.) The original Greek word to "know" is *ginosko* and is defined in *Strong's Exhaustive Concordance of the Bible*, #1097, as " be aware (of), feel, (have) know(-ledge), perceive, be resolved, can speak, be sure, understand."

Do you *know* the truth about God's desire to deliver you from all that tries to control you?

Do you know the truth about the food you eat?

Do you know whether the meat is lean and full of nutrients or full of fat, lacking the vitamins you need?

Do you believe it doesn't matter what you eat? Will you continue to eat sugar and fat-filled foods that lead to death instead of life?

It was true that God wanted to save Israel from Goliath, but the Israelites believed the giant was more powerful than their God. They remained in fear until David exercised his conviction of the truth. And, when he did, they were set free.

David carried five stones to confront Goliath. We have now given you three stones to meditate upon and begin using as weapons against the fat giant who wants to steal and destroy your health.

- *Motivation* will define your purpose.
- *Understanding* will fortify your stance against the enemy.
- *Conviction* will give you the fortitude to fight until the battle is over.

Motivation alone isn't enough to lose weight, although it does contribute to the commitment of finding health. We must add understanding which keeps us from changing our minds. But understanding lacks the action that enforces our diet. So then conviction keeps us fighting until the fat giant is overcome.

> For I know whom I have believed, and am persuaded that he is able to keep that which I have committed unto him against that day.
>
> 2 Timothy 1:12

Are You Convinced of the Truth?

Food Truth #1

We must balance our intake of food with our output of energy.

If we eat too many calories and consume more fat grams than we can use, our body must store the leftover energy somewhere. The body was designed by God to store the extra energy in fat cells. To defeat our giant, we must balance our output of activity with our intake of fuel.

If your activity is not demanding enough to necessitate your consumption, you must cut back. One of my problems was that I saw food as entertainment instead of fuel. Well, my entertainment left me with a lot of excess fuel!

Food Truth #2

Starvation is not balance.

If we withhold food from our body, it is designed to shut down its metabolism and conserve energy to extend its life-span. Our metabolism works better when it is busy digesting low-fat foods than when it shuts down from starvation. Therefore, give your body frequent supplies (five times per day) of low-fat nutritious food to energize it and to stimulate your metabolism.

Food Truth #3

Your body needs four hours of exercise each week.

Balancing exercise with sensible eating keeps the fat giant from rising up against you again. Remember: More food is all right, but it is going to mean more strenuous activity. You would be shocked at how much walking or sit-ups it takes to burn off that fried chicken! After awhile, you will conclude it is not worth it.

Food Truth #4

Believing the truth will save your life, your dream, and your ministry.

Face the facts, believe the truth, and stick to it. The greatest weapon is information, and when you have the truth, do not allow your temptation to dull your convictions. You must have health and energy for anything you want to do with your life. Your strength is dependent on the fuel you feed your body.

Food Truth #5

Spirit-filled living is better than self-control.

If you walk in the Spirit, you will not fulfill the lust of the flesh. (See Galatians 5:16.) Any time we are Spirit-controlled, we are personally empowered.

As believers, we are to become disciples of Jesus Christ. Discipline, which is following the Spirit of God instead of our flesh, brings our behavior into alignment with what we believe in the first place. Balance requires a maturity that overpowers desire.

I am no longer subject to a fleshly king who rules my appetite. I am convinced that eating what is good for my body makes me feel and perform better. I have a peace now, a peace that wasn't present when I faced the bondage of the bulge.

I have conviction that bends my will to choose the truth over the lie. I am convinced that I must control my weight or it will control me. I don't want to take extra luggage with me on my walk through God's abundant life. I am convinced that the taste of French fries is not worth the burden of weight they bring.

Who Is Your King?

The story of the fat King Eglon in the third chapter of Judges fascinates me. A new generation of Israelites were tested to see whether they would obey the Lord's commands which were given to their forefathers through Moses. This young generation had never had to fight for anything like their forefathers had. It seems fair to say, they were immature and self-indulgent.

They did evil in the sight of the Lord by serving other gods, so He left them until they cried out for deliverance. In His mercy he gave them a king who kept them in peace for forty years. Then, once again, they became selfish and did evil in the sight of the Lord, so the Lord gave Eglon power over the people of Israel. Eglon took possession of their city and ruled them for eighteen years.

The children of Israel cried out for help again, and God sent Ehud, a left-handed man to Eglon. He came with a double-edged sword about a foot and a half long and told Eglon he had a message for him from God. As Eglon rose from his seat, Ehud plunged the sword into the king's belly.

The king was so fat, the entire sword disappeared in his gut! Even the handle sank in as the sword came out the back. Verse 22 says that Ehud could not withdraw the sword, and dirt came out of King Eglon. What a disgusting sight that must have been!

Don't dig your grave with a knife and fork.

— English Proverb

Ehud escaped and later returned with the children of Israel to fight the men of Moab. These robust men of valor slew ten thousand, so that not one of Moab's men were left. They beheaded their giant and remained in peace for eighty years.

How Long Have You Been in Bondage?

Eighteen years of bondage was a long time for the Israelites to be oppressed before they were willing to fight for freedom. How long are you willing to submit to the lusty king before you are ready to fight for your right to peace?

Jesus, the King of Peace, stands ready with the sword of the Spirit, which is the Word of God, to impale your enemy with truth. That's why it is so important that you include the Word of God in your fight. It is God's Word that gives you the power to slay the giant and let all the dirt, candy, pies, and greasy foods spill out of your life.

The truth is that too many pizzas, cookies, and cobblers really can kill us. But before taking our lives, they will destroy our zeal and enthusiasm for the work of God. We need to let the truth cut away our deception and drain the dirt out of our diet.

Exercise — Spirit, Mind, and Body

Fight the enemy by exercising your body. Go for a walk, get on a tread mill, or take your kids swimming. Get some sunshine! Remember what I said earlier: You will never be younger than you are today, so there will never be a better time to begin than right now.

Your body appreciates with use. God didn't make your body to wear out with use, like the cars and appliances that depreciate in a few years. God made your body to become stronger and healthier the more you use it.

Fight the enemy by exercising your mind. Listen to motivational and inspirational tapes while you walk. Watch edifying videos while you keep pace on a treadmill. Expand your knowledge to increase the mental warfare against the enemy.

Fight the enemy by exercising your faith. Faith comes by hearing the Word of God. Hold onto truth and don't be immature as those described in Hebrews 5:12 who need to be taught again and again the elementary truths of God's Word. Be convinced of the Word of God and win your victories by your conviction of truth.

Excuse me for slightly paraphrasing Hebrews 5:12 and 13, but these verses express our point well, "Get away from milk and start eating solid food! Anyone who lives on milk (and cookies) is still an infant, and is not acquainted with the teaching of righteousness. Solid food is for the mature, who by reason of use have their senses exercised to discern both good and evil."

Strength of body, mind, and spirit increase with use. Learn to discern good food from bad food. Sure, everything is permitted, but not everything is good for us. It is good to mature in our ability to make choices that lead to life.

The next time you are at the sub-shop and the sandwich maker asks you, "Would that be with cheese?" say, "No, thank you!"

The next time some pointless TV program invites you to linger a little longer say, "No, I'm taking a walk and listening to the Word of God on my tape player for the next hour."

The next time your faith begins to weaken and cause you to doubt God's deliverance from your enemy, say, "No, I will not doubt the Lord Who delivered David from Goliath and Israel from fat, self-indulgent kings who took their possessions. God is here to deliver me too."

Many of us are carrying too much baggage with us to truly enjoy the life we are living. Travel is more fun when we can fit everything we need in a small overnight bag.

Remember when our children were babies and we had to take toys, diaper bags, strollers, and cribs with us everywhere we went? Weight that attaches to our body is much the same as all the extra baggage that is needed for infants. Cumbersome weight distracts from the pleasure of the trip.

Excessive weight also distracts people when we meet them. Instead of noticing who we are on the inside, all they see is these packages and pockets of fat we are carrying.

Have you ever sat on a plane and had a large person squeeze by you? They almost dislocate your shoulder with their hips. They might be a nice person, but that is not what you remember about them.

As we mature in our ability to make disciplined choices about what we eat, our pleasure in life increases. Our confidence increases when we are in public.

Make choices from your knowledge of truth. Don't default to ignorance. Read the labels on the food you eat. Be truthful about the portions you are eating and respect the amount of fat grams you consume. If there are 19 grams of fat in 1 ounce of ranch dressing, don't add two ladles full on your baked potato and salad and call it even for the day. Dressing can add 60 grams of fat to an otherwise healthy meal.

If you have ever met people and watched to catch their reaction to your weight, checking to see if they were smirking or staring, you know that this battle is worth fighting.

It is worth fighting to get your dignity back. And you are going to win if you know the truth and depend on your conviction when you need strength to resist temptation.

chapter 7

Don't Forget Your Bag of River Stones!

A slingshot is a useless weapon without stones.

Faith is useless without the knowledge of God's truth. Knowledge of how to do something is easily achieved, but truth reveals why it should be done. For example, David had knowledge of how to use a slingshot. But his faith was bigger than Goliath because he also knew the truth — why God wanted the giant destroyed.

David knew God had the ability to deliver Israel because He had delivered his forefathers from Egypt. So David's faith for his own need was great because he knew this truth: God wanted to keep his generation from becoming slaves to the Philistines. David also knew Israel's freedom glorified God and that when the Gentiles saw the blessing of God on His people, they would hunger for the God of Israel.

Likewise, knowledge of how to lose weight is good. And knowledge of the truth about why we should be fit will empower our faith. But our freedom from the bondage of a heavy burden glorifies God.

That's why I wanted to write this book. There are many books that give the facts about dieting and the importance of maintaining an ideal weight, but facts cannot always reveal the truth, which simplifies our purpose, reason, and motive.

Truth sparkles with clarity and brings refreshment to those who receive it. Jesus spoke with great simplicity when He said, "I am the way, the truth, and the life: no man cometh unto the Father, but by me" (John 14:6).

I have learned to seek truth when the enemy pursues me. Freedom comes through knowledge of the truth, which always provides an escape to safety. The Lord promised, "If ye continue in my word, then are ye my disciples indeed; And ye shall know the truth, and the truth shall make you free" (John 8:31,32).

> God is more glorified by living sacrifices than by prematurely dead saints.

By knowing truth, we discern the larger picture, which brings understanding and conviction. When we understand God's motive for making our bodies the way He did, our knowledge can set us free to enjoy His design by working *with* His plan for us instead of *against* it.

When we have knowledge of why God wants us to be healthy, we become passionate in our pursuit of fitness. When we have knowledge of what is making us burdened with weight, we have power to lay that weight aside.

We were created to live forever. Even though our bodies age and eventually die, we still have the original design God gave us for surviving eternity. Our body knows many ways to protect itself. If we cut ourselves, the blood coagulates and forms a natural bandage. If we starve ourselves, our metabolism slows down to preserve fuel for future use.

When the metabolism slows down, dieters begin to complain and say, "I just don't understand, I'm hardly eating anything at all and I can't lose weight." But the truth is, God didn't intend for you to starve. Your metabolism will remain more active and burn more calories if it is busy digesting five small low-fat meals instead of one meager meal each day.

Your body has to be recalibrated once you lose the weight. It must accept this new and right you. That will take a little time, so you must know that your body will try to fight the new rules for awhile, because it is trying to protect you.

I worshiped God when I realized He designed my body to store food for survival. Then I repented when I realized I had abused my body through excesses and inactivity. I had literally confused my body. I had to reprogram it before it broke down from too much weight.

My poor body was stretching its skin and building new drawers to try to find a place to dump all the junk I was piling in it. When I quit abusing it, the poor thing thought something was wrong. My body was the victim of food abuse!

I didn't know I was abusing it. I didn't know how I should eat. But I do have to tell you that when people say, "What you don't know can't hurt you," that is not the truth. What you don't know can kill you! I just thank God that the new healthy way of eating gave my body healing and restoration before it gave up in exasperation and died!

Knowledge Is the Fourth Stone

Many people don't *know* the truth about their body's survival system or how the food they eat affects their energy. Most people don't know the truth about the content of the food they are eating. They don't know if their meal is full of fat or is vitamin deficient.

You can gain knowledge of the truth simply by reading the nutrition labels on the food you buy. You can also gain knowledge by asking waiters and chefs in restaurants how many calories and fat grams are in the food they serve you. Many food establishments have printed menus with calorie and fat-gram calculations for those who ask for the truth.

Knowledge of how many fat grams are in the foods you eat will give you the conviction you need to make healthy choices. You can know when you have had enough calories for the day. Choose the foods you eat by what you *know* to be true, not by what you *think* is true.

You will be surprised at the truth of what is in some of your favorite foods. You will find that the bread pudding you think is your enemy only has seven grams of fat. The salad, which you thought was good for you, is actually full of 56 grams of fat by the time you put four helpings of dressing on your otherwise healthy greens.

Start With a Visit to Your Doctor

The guidelines presented here are for healthy people who simply want to learn to balance and manage their lifestyles. I want to clearly establish in this book that you need to get a check-up from your doctor and let him know you want to lose weight.

If you are sick and have health problems, you should not try to lose weight unless your physician has told you to do so and is actively involved with your plan.

The skills I am sharing are merely testimonial in nature. They are based on standard health rules and my personal experience, which restored my body and enhanced my walk with God. If you have special needs and concerns, always seek the counsel of your physician. Then use the scriptures I have suggested to encourage you in the program that your doctor designed for you. Here are some tips that are universally effective.

During your initial attack against your weight, you will need to eat fewer calories and take in fewer fat grams. When you reach your normal body size, you will need to increase your calories and fat-gram intake to maintain the weight you become.

> And Jesus answered him, saying, It is written, That man shall not live by bread alone, but by every word of God.
>
> Luke 4:4

Your doctor will tell you what those counts should be for your level of activity, age, and height. Please understand, we are not wanting to present this book as a diet book, but as a balanced lifestyle teaching that leads to a better way of life.

I simply want to pass on to you the truths that worked for me, as well as some tips for the body and low-fat recipes from Carlo. For that reason, we will avoid stating how many calories and how many fat grams you should have. There are too many variables for us to try to make such a calculation. Your doctor will supply that information.

I want to give you some basic tools of knowledge you can apply to any weight-loss program. Many diets give you methods to pull off weight, but they don't impart knowledge so you can understand how to maintain the loss.

Most weight-loss programs want you to be dependent on their food sources so you will continue to buy their program. True knowledge will give you the power to make choices without depending on someone else to dictate what you should or shouldn't eat.

Weight control is simple math. If you eat more calories and fat than you need, you will become overweight. And if you don't eat enough, you will be underweight. But if you balance your intake of food and output of energy, you will become and maintain the size your body frame was designed to carry.

After establishing how many calories and fat grams you should eat each day, the next step is to keep an honest record of how much you are eating. Refer to the label or to a nutrition guide for details of calorie counts. Keep an accurate assessment of the portions you are eating so you will know when you truly have had enough food for the day.

There are many calorie counters in the health and nutrition section of your local bookstore. One I think is especially convenient is a pocket-sized edition called *The T-Factor Fat Gram Counter.* If you can't locate the guide, you can write to the attention of the Special Sales Department, W. W. Norton & Company, Inc., 500 Fifth Avenue, New York, NY 10110. They have two other handy references titled, *The Low-Fat Fast Food Guide – How To Eat Right When You're Eating Out,* and *The Low-Fat Supermarket Shopper's Guide.*

Be Mentally Prepared

At least two weeks before you start to count calories and fat grams, begin mentally preparing for the change of lifestyle you desire. Take time to experience the pleasure of getting outside and exercising your body. Use the exercise time to think about what you really want to happen with your life.

For instance, if you want to lose weight, establish your motivation to lose weight. Find a reason that will hold you on your path, as we discussed in chapter 4.

Solidify in your understanding that the active life you want to live is dependent on the food you choose to eat. Examine your life to see if there are ways you can simplify your routine to make time for exercise and better meal planning.

Continue to ask yourself if your long-term achievement will be worth the short-term sacrifice that may be required. Busy people who won't put their health above their activities are not convicted of the need for the changes that will bring about their victory.

Change will come more quickly for those who are ready to follow their new eating pattern at least 90 percent of the time. And remember any healthy person can follow these truths that I used to lay aside the weight and enjoy my dream.

Exercise Your Spiritual Power

The second phase of laying aside the weight, after mental preparation, involves restricting your intake of food for a period of time. In addition to lowering your fat gram and calorie intake, you can add fasting to your lifestyle. Fasting will enhance your body's ability to digest and process foods. If you put spirit over flesh, you will always have success.

Carlo explains in his tips for healthy living at the back of this book how a routine fast every other week for twenty-four to thirty-six hours is very healthy for your body. During this time you should only drink liquids such as 100 percent fruit juices or caffeine-free herbal teas.

Never starve yourself. Even when fasting, make certain you are drinking tea or juice at regular intervals. If you don't eat or drink regularly, your body's starvation defenses will kick in, lowering your metabolism and storing, instead of burning, fat.

Burning up 3000 calories uses a pound of body weight. So two fasts each month saves you 1500 calories each day, or a total of 3000 calories. A fast can help you slim down as well as give your body an opportunity to eliminate toxins which pull down your energy level.

Many people are discovering the pleasure of fasting and are renewing the biblical observance of using the day of fasting to pray and seek direction from the Lord. Fasting improves your willpower and self-control. Fasting enhances your physical senses and brings clarity to your thought processes. You will be surprised at how quickly the giant within you is quieted by a true fast. You may also be surprised by how little nourishment the child within you truly needs to be satisfied.

During a fast, drink as much water as you can with teas and juices. The best juices are pineapple, grapefruit, and orange juice. Every time you are wanting something to eat, you can sip these clear liquids.

An example of a thirty-six hour fast: Begin after the evening meal on Thursday night, drink juice all day Friday, then break the fast on Saturday morning by eating fruit. Wait thirty minutes, and resume your regular diet for another two weeks before fasting again.

M-m-m-m, Breakfast!

Breakfast is the most important meal of the day, but it's also very difficult to find healthy breakfast foods. So Carlo has some wonderful breakfast recipes in this book. His crepes are delicious. You won't believe how good you can eat while still reaching your ideal weight.

We eat turkey kielbasa for breakfast. When traveling, we ask for turkey slices for breakfast food. If you have them, grill the turkey slices. It is very similar to grilled ham but with far less fat grams. Many restaurants have turkey in their kitchen even if it doesn't show on the breakfast menu.

Eggbeaters, or egg substitutes, make great omelets. You can add all types of vegetables and fat-free cheeses. You can even make a ham and cheese omelet with low-fat ham. It's really, really good.

My wife prefers egg whites instead of egg substitutes, so Carlo puts a little bit of yellow food coloring in her omelet. You really can't tell the difference in the taste, but the coloring enhances its "psychological value." We even make fat-free biscuits. It's a little more work, but worth the taste and the "end" result!

We also eat a lot of potatoes. We add onions and peppers, but we steam them instead of fry them like we used to. As you know, we're southern people, so we do grits real well — without butter. There's a new butter spray that tastes great but doesn't have any fat grams in it, so many of our favorite dishes can still taste like good southern meals.

You can actually eat regular eggs since they only have about six grams of fat in them, but I choose to use the fat somewhere else. Because I know how to alleviate fat from one place, I can use it in another. I would rather do Eggbeaters and have a "piece" of Danish later. Incidentally, there are some very tasty fat-free Danish pastries that are available in most grocery stores. They are delicious and you will not even notice they are fat-free.

Please Sir, May I Have Less?

(Or for fun we could say, "Fe, fi, fo fum, don't put mayo on my bun!)

The main thing I have to fight when I travel is food. Some of the better restaurants have healthy cuisine, but a lot of them do not. When they don't have a light menu, you have to create an entree by talking to the chef.

Just tell him you want the chicken breast, but don't want it cooked in butter or covered afterward with butter or sauces. If it says *creamy*, it means it's milk-based and it's going to have lots of fat or cheese in it. I avoid those choices.

When I go to a seafood restaurant, for instance, I ask them to make me a special toasted bread. I don't eat their little cheese breads, even though I love them. Though they only have seven grams of fat in each biscuit, I used to eat about ten of them!

When I know I can't stop eating something, I've learned not to even start. I get the broiled fish and instead of a baked potato I sometimes get the rice. Some places put butter and oils in the rice, so the baked potato is often a better choice if you leave off the toppings.

> Knowledge can make a difference at the breakfast bar. Did you realize that one medium Danish pastry has 19 grams of fat? A cinnamon raisin bagel has 2 grams of fat and some English muffins less than 1 gram of fat?

I learned to eat baked potatoes without butter. It's good when I mash it up and put salt and pepper on it. It's really not bad, but *you* have to want to do this. If *you* get into it, after awhile you will be eager to get back on the routine if you get off of it.

When we spent a holiday in Cancun, Mexico, we ate whatever we wanted, but we still didn't eat crazy stuff. We did eat things that we hadn't had in over a year — after all, we were on vacation. But coming back to our routine was not like I thought it would be. I was ready to go back to it because it doesn't bother me. I like the way I feel when I eat healthy food.

I try to make healthy choices. Creamed spinach is worse than regular spinach. Milk-based lobster bisque and clam chowder isn't as good for us as vegetable soup or chicken noodle soup. Some foods I am careful to keep to a minimum or avoid completely, such as milk, cheese, sauces, butters, oils, and fried foods. The only pork I now eat is fat-free ham.

Exercise Your Body

The best way to burn calories and drop the weight is still exercise. As you lose weight, your body has to adapt to its new size. As I said before, my wife can eat less food and lose weight without as much exercise. But I still want the food, so I pay the price on the treadmill. My trick to enduring the treadmill is to watch an action movie while I walk. That really works for me because the more action it has, the faster I walk.

I actually forget I'm on the treadmill because I become one of those people in the movie. Sometimes music is a nice distraction. Other times I use my exercise time as a

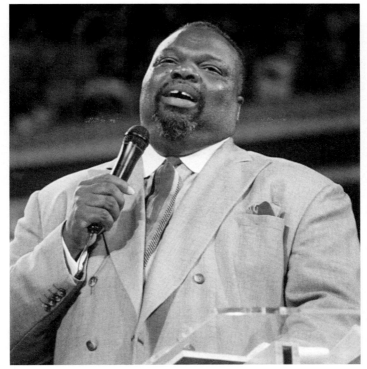

Bishop T. D. Jakes preaching at the Manpower Conference
in 1995. (330 pounds)

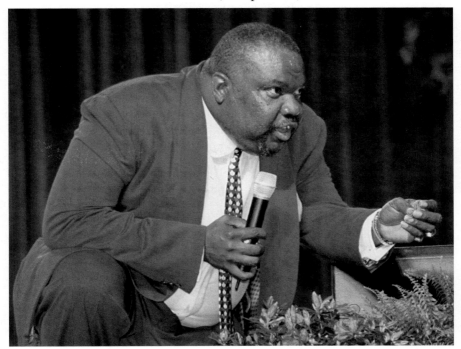

Bishop T. D. Jakes preaching at the Singles Conference in
Indianapolis, Indiana, in September of 1996.   (338 pounds)

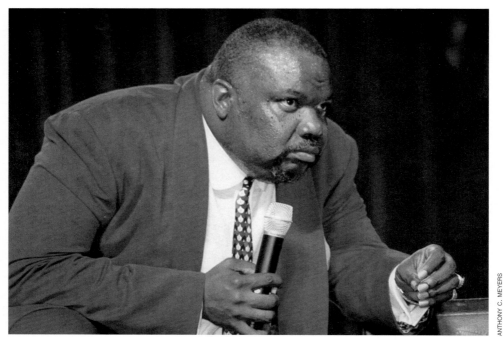

Bishop T. D. Jakes preaching at the Singles Conference in Indianapolis, Indiana, in September of 1996. (338 pounds)

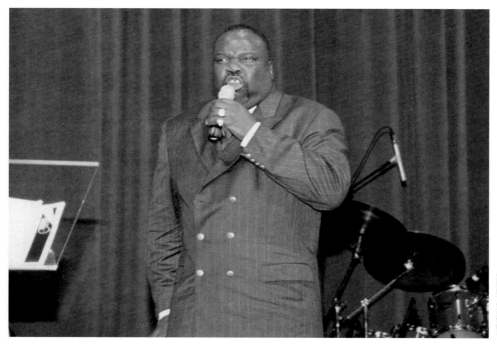

Bishop T. D. Jakes preaching at the Manpower Conference in Los Angeles, California, in 1996. (320 pounds)

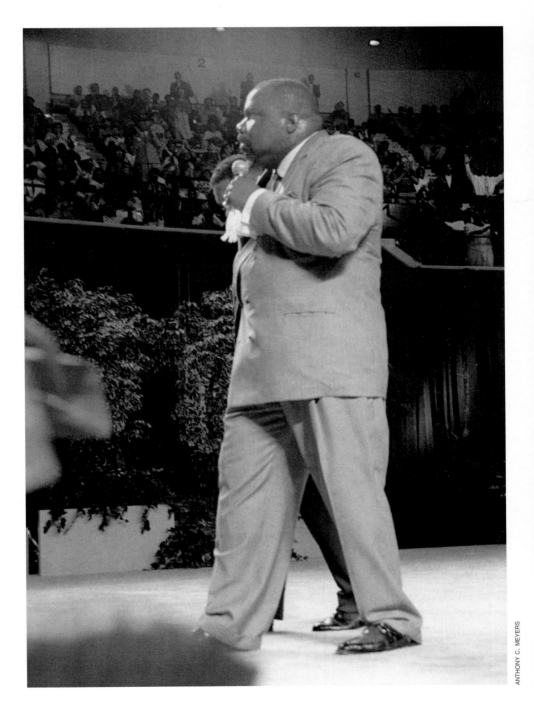

Bishop T. D. Jakes preaching in Tampa, Florida, in 1996. (290 pounds)

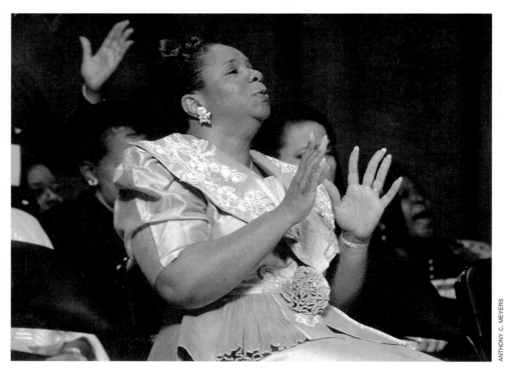

Serita Jakes at the Woman, Thou Art Loosed Conference in New Orleans,
Louisiana, in 1996. (210 pounds)

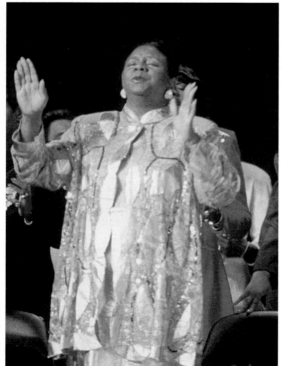

Serita Jakes at the Woman,
Thou Art Loosed Conference
in New Orleans, Louisiana, in
1996. (210 pounds)

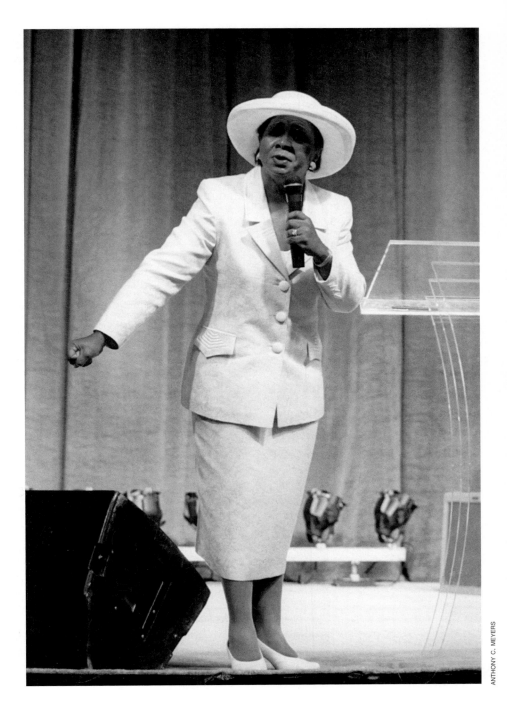

Serita Jakes speaking in Chicago, Illinois, in 1997. (169 pounds)

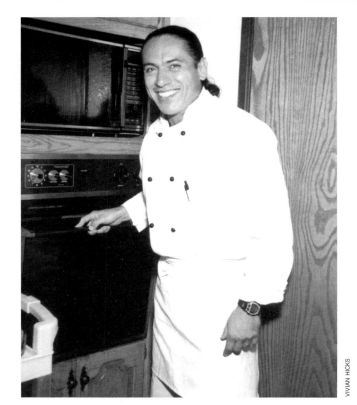

Carlo Gabrelian
practices what he
preaches – eating
low-fat foods and
exercising daily.
September 1997

VIVIAN HICKS

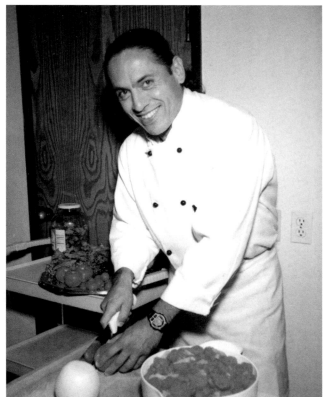

Nutritionist Carlo
Gabrelian, prepares
delicious, low-fat foods
for Bishop and
Mrs. T. D. Jakes.
September 1997

VIVIAN HICKS

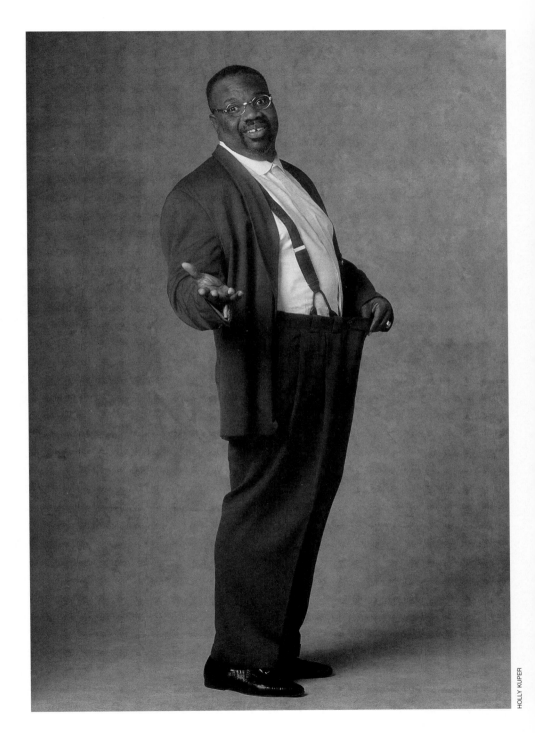

Bishop T. D. Jakes pictured in the same suit as on the first page
of this photo section! (228 pounds)

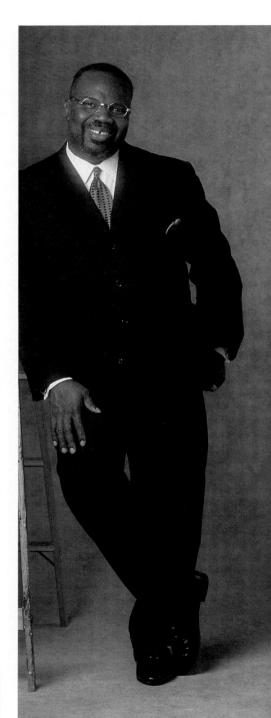

This photo of Bishop
T. D. Jakes was taken
in September of 1997
after losing 100
pounds!
(228 pounds)

time to clear my head and meditate in prayer. When you are busy, you have to learn to combine activities.

The action movies are enjoyable, especially if you are like I am when I do get to watch something entertaining. My wife watches me watch the movies, because I'm running to help the good guy saying, "Kill 'em." I'm one of those guys who jumps on top of the end table yelling, "Watch out! watch out! Don't let him go!"

When you take that kind of energy and put it on the treadmill...well, the results are effective. I'm high energy, so the hour passes much more quickly when something exciting is there for me to watch.

I didn't always walk fast on the treadmill. I was so overweight at first, it seemed unwise to go from being completely sedentary to trying to act like I was some physical education major. Even now, there are those who go faster, but remember, this is not a competition!

Whatever speed you go will be faster than sitting in that chair eating buttered popcorn all day. Then, once I was used to one speed, I went to the next. You want to be challenged by your workout, not murdered by it.

Now I start out at about three miles an hour. I do that for about ten or fifteen minutes, then I kick it up to four miles an hour for another ten or fifteen minutes. At the peak, I walk about six miles an hour for about ten minutes. By then I'm sweaty and ready to slow back down to four miles an hour for the rest of the hour.

Okay, I admit, at the end of an hour, I'm through! I fall off of it and think, *Uh-h-h-hh, thank You, Lord.*

When I first started, I walked the speed of two miles an hour, which is fairly slow. I was so overweight, I didn't want to have a heart attack on the thing. My heart would have said, "That's it, I quit." And I didn't start out doing an hour. At the very beginning I did fifteen minutes, then thirty, then I walked an hour every other day, which is better than thirty minutes daily. Once your heart rate is up over thirty minutes, everything over thirty minutes burns pre-existing fat.

I had to work my weight down gradually with a system, but a lot of my success was the exercise. I am faithful to my machine. But whatever exercise you choose, just keep doing it and get better at it. It is an absolute necessity for balance in your life.

Reduce the risk of dehydration by drinking water before you feel thirsty, especially if you're working out. Drinking a glass of water fifteen minutes before you start a workout is a good practice to follow.

Sam Grossman

If you find something that you like or you don't mind doing, it's a lot better. Walking is something I enjoy, so I just step on the machine and take off. My wife does better on a rowing machine you sit on and pull back and forth.

When I travel, I don't exercise as faithfully as I do at home, but I still try to get down to the hotel gym and work out a little bit. It's best to have something you can do in the privacy of your own room. If it's convenient, you will stick to it better. It can be an obstacle if you have to get dressed up to go sweat in public.

To make every phase work, knowing the truth is your most powerful weapon for casting aside the weight. When you know how to balance your food and find the right exercise to keep your body strong and youthful, you won't be dependent on dieting programs ever again.

chapter 8

Don't Stop Now, Behead the Giant

Never trust a wounded enemy.

David knew that the only good enemy is a defeated one. With a slingshot and sword, David slew Goliath and secured his future against the giant's threats of bondage. Through his obedience to God's plan for his life, David set a nation free to enjoy God's grace.

Before meeting Goliath, David had seen God deliver him from smaller enemies. Then, his opponents grew larger, he saw that God's power proved to be unchanging. By the time he faced this giant, he could boldly declare, "The Lord that delivered me out of the paw of the lion, and out of the paw of the bear, he will deliver me out of the hand of this Philistine." (1 Samuel 17:37).

David had a powerful perspective on the problem. His motivation to see the Israelites set free was greater than his temptation to run away from the enemy. David understood the big picture and he didn't want to be a slave to the Philistines. He was convinced that faith in God would bring deliverance for his family and nation. David had knowledge of God's unfailing power, and trusted that his obedience to God would get results.

Trust Is the Fifth Stone

David's trust was in God. Knowing that he needed no other shield of protection, David laid aside the weight of Saul's armor and marched to war with weapons he could trust from previous experience. Saul wanted David to wear a bronze helmet and a coat of mail, but David took them off.

What weapons are you using against your giant? The five symbolic stones of *motivation, understanding, conviction, knowledge,* and *trust* I have given you WILL defeat your enemy. I call this "transferable truth," which you can always carry with you into future battles. Keep your slingshot of power, which is faith in God, and arm yourself with the following stones to prepare yourself for your next war.

STONE #1: Be motivated by the truth of God's plan for you.

STONE #2: Understand that your actions expedite His plan.

STONE #3: Be convinced of God's victorious power.

STONE #4: Act on the knowledge of the truth.

STONE #5: Trust that your obedience to God will get results.

God wants you to enjoy the abundant life, which includes good health. We glorify Him through our life, not through a premature death as a result of poor living habits.

Since the time you first believed on Jesus Christ as your personal Savior, how many times have you seen Him

> The only way to change one's body weight is to begin a life-long series of new habits. But the notion of going on some radical diet for a while and then stopping is a waste of time.
>
> — Dr. Jules Hirsch

deliver you? Do you believe that an eating disorder is more difficult for God than the changes you have already seen Him perform in your life? God's own Son bore your sickness and infirmities, so God wants you to enjoy health. Trust that your obedience to God will bring results.

In Whom Have You Put Your Trust?

Have other people tried to arm you with weight-loss programs that have only brought you into more bondage? Some programs can keep you so preoccupied with what you are eating that you can't think of anything else. You are not free as long as someone else is deciding what you should eat. You need to *know* what is good for you and what isn't, so you are in control of your own health. Knowing the truth will set you free.

Many diet plans and weight-loss programs succeed through your dependence on them. They want you to keep coming back to them so they can sell you their literature and food.

But if you understand the food process, you can ultimately become independent of pre-measured, processed foods. When you have knowledge, you are able to enter a grocery store or restaurant and make intelligent choices that are good for you.

When you understand how your body operates, you can maintain your ideal weight without paying a program fee. Unfortunately, most of us know very little about the body we live within.

For example, I never understood food as fuel or associated its value in terms of having enough energy for my performance. I saw food as a pleasure or stress breaker. I saw it as everything but fuel. And I never understood the practical design of my body. All I knew was, an isolated event of giving up a second helping wasn't going to make me drop the pounds, so I went ahead and ate it.

Now I understand that while an isolated sacrifice does not make much difference, a lifestyle committed to eating healthy food and exercising my body does impact the way I feel and what I am able to enjoy. God always gives you something to pull you out of a trap. Even though you might be overweight and out of shape physically, you can be in shape spiritually and mentally. You can use your strengths to defend your weakest parts.

There comes a point at the end of various diets, pills, stomach stapling, and numerous crazy attempts at weight loss that you finally say, "If there's going to be any hope for me at all, Jesus, You're going to have to do it." When you commit your giant to prayer, the devil gets terrified. When you release the gifts of the Spirit and engage spiritual warfare against a physical problem, you get to the root of the issue. Wouldn't it be great if we all had prayed a little sooner, before all the suffering?

Bartimaeus sat beside the highway because he had adopted a lifestyle of begging in order to survive his condition of blindness. You can read his story in Mark 10:46-52. Anytime we have a condition we think will not change, we adapt everything to accommodate it, from the way we dress to where we sit to the size of our furniture. But Bartimaeus heard that Jesus was passing by, and even though he had lost his eyes, he had not lost his ears.

Bartimaeus used his hearing to fight for his eyesight. He listened for a way out of his darkness and he heard that Jesus was passing by. The Bible says he cried out, "Jesus, thou son of David, have mercy on me." The Amplified Bible adds, "Have mercy on me NOW!" He called out to the Lord because he knew that if there were going to be any changes in his life, God was going to have to do it.

Bartimaeus cried out so much, it irritated people around him. Many censured him severely, telling him to keep still, but he just called out all the more, "Jesus, thou son of David, have mercy on me." He did not stop calling for Jesus until he got the His attention. Bartimaeus called the name of the Lord until Jesus stood still. Then, when Jesus called to him, Bartimaeus laid aside his coat and ran to Him.

That coat identified Bartimaeus as a beggar. It was his source of survival. He wore it because he had expected to remain on the side of the road, where he could beg for money and food. But when Bartimaeus heard the voice of the Lord, he suddenly knew he wouldn't need his beggar's coat anymore.

> And Jesus said unto him, Go thy way; thy faith hath made thee whole.
>
> Mark 10:52

He threw off his coat and leaped up. This was his way of proclaiming, "I'm not ever gonna' need this beggar's coat again. The Lord has called my name, and I am no longer in need of begging for food. This coat no longer identifies who I am."

Bartimaeus knew the truth before there was evidence of the victory. Notice how the five weapons worked for him against his blindness. He was *motivated* by the hope of being a full-sighted individual. He *understood* that responding to the voice of the Lord was going to set him free. He was *convinced* the Lord wanted him to see. He had *knowledge* that God was able to heal him, because he had heard about so many others who had been healed by Jesus. And, Bartimaeus *trusted* that his obedience in responding to the voice of the Lord would get him the results he was after.

Jesus said, "Go your way; your faith has healed you." Bartimaeus immediately received his sight and walked with Jesus on the road.

Did you know that the Bible says, "Ye have not, because ye ask not" (James 4:2). Jesus said that whatever we ask in His name He will do it. (See John 14:13.) The word "ask" used in this context is the Greek word *aiteo*, which means "to beg, call for, crave, desire, and require." (*Strong's Concordance*, #154.)

Have you begged God for help with your weight? Has your desire to be at your ideal body weight been so evident that your craving for health has consumed your prayer life?

When God gives us the grace to change, we can lay aside the weight, the beggar's coat, and the provisions we have made to hide the condition we were in. We can stop wearing topcoats in August. We can leap up and come out of hiding. We can quit wearing drab colors all the time. We can feel good about ourselves, because we don't expect to sit on the sidelines again.

For me, laying aside my garment was getting rid of the clothes I didn't expect to wear again. It was an act of faith to say, "I'm not going to come back to this place."

The tempter mocked, "Suppose you gain weight again. You're going to need that suit someday." But I gave away the coat, because the truth had set me free. Somebody else can have it, but I would rather they have these five stones of truth. Then we could just burn the oversized coat!

My faith refreshes me, and God has given me weapons to keep me armed for future battles:

- I am motivated to enjoy the abundant life.
- I understand that healthy food energizes God's plan for my life.
- I have conviction that God will help me.
- I have knowledge about food that I didn't have before.
- I trust that my obedience to eat right will have godly results.

I'm not going to need that big coat anymore! I am going to wear short sleeves in the summer. Bartimaeus laid aside his coat, because he knew he wasn't going to be blind again. He left the coat lying in the place where he used to sit. When people walked past his old spot on the road, people probably said, "Whose coat is that?"

"Well that belonged to the blind beggar who used to sit there."

"Where is he now?"

"I don't know, but I do know that he's not blind anymore."

Our greatest testimony is that big, old coat we leave behind. I can point to it and say, "That used to be me, but now I'm free."

You Can Dance When the War is Over!

I now enjoy the victory of the battle. My body has adapted to my new weight, and I don't have to struggle so much to keep the weight off. My habits have changed, and my lifestyle contributes to the success I have achieved in my new body weight. Coming home from our recent vacation in Cancun was a real litmus test for me. The food was delicious.

I like seafood, and I was able to pick out the fresh fish and have it cooked however I wanted. We had incredible meals, and I ate things I had given up while trying to lose weight. But now I am able to increase my calories in order to maintain my ideal weight.

> If you are going to a restaurant, determine before you get there what you will and will not eat. Let the truth guide your decisions, not the smell of fried foods!

I had a chopped lobster dish I will never forget. It was filled with mushrooms and covered with a bernaise sauce. There was time during my battle to lose weight that, if I had eaten like we did on our trip, I would have easily gained twelve pounds in a week. I didn't get on the scales, but I could tell by the way my clothes were fitting each day that I was doing fine. I knew I wasn't in the war zone anymore.

Carlo says that after six months of maintaining your ideal weight, your body will adapt and you won't have to fight the battle so hard. I am happy to say it gets easier, but you should celebrate as you go. Don't wait until you are your ideal weight to be happy about the progress you are making. Celebrate when you say "No cheese, please" on your next taco.

Celebrate when you lose ten pounds, even if you have ninety pounds to go. Rejoice when you make it outdoors for a walk even if you missed the day before. God didn't create the earth in one day, but He continued to stop and say, "It is good." He celebrated each phase of progress in His plan.

When you celebrate, find ways to reward yourself without eating something you shouldn't. Be careful if you celebrate by going to a movie. That concession stand is a real health hazard for obesity-prone movie viewers! When you go through that enemy battlefield, I recommend you wear camouflage fatigues and just crawl through like Rambo, with your machete between your teeth. Don't give in to the cheese-covered nachos and greasy popcorn. Even yogurt-covered peanuts have 26 grams of fat in a one-half cup serving!

I find it depressing when I do something against my better judgment, so I take my own low-fat food to parties. It keeps me from a relapse into my old bad habits. Sometimes you have to nibble on something to keep others from feeling like you have broken fellowship. Our society is food-oriented, and some people make you feel like you haven't celebrated until you "break bread" together.

I used to fear I would just start blowing up. Perhaps you have seen the movie, *The Nutty Professor*. Eddie Murphy plays the part of a fat man who drinks a wonder drug and loses all of his extra weight. But when the chemical wears off, his lips suddenly *pop* out as his body expands to its obese origins. His face triples in size, and his fingers suddenly bulge beyond their natural limits. It's so funny, because I thought I was going to suffer the Nutty Professor syndrome too. It can be a big fear. I almost didn't write the book because of it.

I dreaded the thought of writing this book and then bursting out like the Nutty Professor, but I wrote the book anyway. I wanted to make a statement. To be honest, I am telling this story to lock myself into the victory. It will remind me of how great I feel about winning this battle. Like David, my victory isn't just for me anymore. And your victory will bless many people who want you to stay around to enjoy a long and healthy life.

Revelation 12:10 says that the people overcame the accuser of the brethren by the blood of the Lamb and the word of their testimony. You must speak about your victories. Many people don't understand how powerful words are. Proverbs 18:21 says, "Death and life are in the power of the tongue: and they that love it shall eat the fruit thereof." Talking about your victories keeps the joy you feel alive. Jesus said in Mark 11:23 that you would have whatever you *say:*

> "For verily I say unto you, That whosoever shall say unto this mountain, Be thou removed, and be thou cast into the sea; and shall not doubt in his heart, but shall believe that those things which he saith shall come to pass; he shall have whatsoever he saith."
>
> Mark 11:23

Celebrate your victories by affirming yourself, appreciating yourself, speaking well of yourself, and feeling good about your accomplishments. One of the greatest ways to celebrate is to talk about your success with your family and friends. It reinforces your faith, which comes by hearing and hearing by the Word of God. (See Romans 10.17.)

When you hear yourself say, "This is how I live now, and this is what I do," it reaffirms the truth of it in you. First John 5:4 says, "This is the victory that overcometh the world, even our faith." In speaking our faith we build ourselves up, which is the purpose and process of Christianity.

Hebrews 10:25 stresses the importance of assembling together to urge one another to be strengthened and built up by what we believe. It is difficult to eat unhealthy food when you see how encouraged people are by your success in something they also desire. Accountability helps you to stay victorious.

Surround yourself with positive people who affirm you and celebrate you. Find people who build your confidence and who rally beside you and say, "Oh, my you look wonderful! You're doing so good."

Trust Will Keep Your Victory

Once you win the war of weight, there may be other battles, but you won't have to fight the same enemy again. You can trust God for lasting results. Maintenence is trusting Him on a day-to-day basis. I believe you will discover, like I did, that new battles are easier because your faith increases after each new victory. The enemy may try to send new anxieties to steal your con-

> A sound mind in a sound body is a short but full description of a happy state in this World. He that has these two has little more to wish for; and he that wants either of them will be little the better for anything else.
>
> John Locke

fidence, because he wants you to recant your position in fear of a new giant. This is where trust becomes your final weapon against the devil.

Goliath had some relatives that were as big as he was. The story is told beginning in 2 Samuel 21:16 that many years later David tried to fight another Philistine giant, but he became faint. His men killed the giant and swore to him, saying in verse 17, "Thou shalt go no more out with us to battle, that thou quench not the light of Israel." They were saying that his life was valuable to them, so he never fought giants again. His earlier victories had won him the right to rest from the battle.

David had to learn to trust God to provide deliverance from the giants. It was clear God didn't want David to be a martyr for Israel. He wanted David to be a living sacrifice to bear His glory to the nation of God. God wants us alive for His glory too.

Hebrews 4 explains that God wants us to enter His full and complete rest reserved for His people. When we learn to trust God for our battles, we enter into the rest He wants us to enjoy. James 2:17 says that faith without works is dead. But when faith graduates it becomes trust. When we move to a level of trust in God, we can enjoy the fruit of our labor and relax in full assurance of God's ever-present grace.

David spoke to the Lord the day He delivered him from the hands of all his enemies saying, "The Lord is my Rock and my Fortress and my Deliverer. My God, my Rock, in Him will I take refuge; my Shield and the Horn of my salvation; my Stronghold and my Refuge, my Savior — You save me from violence. I call on the Lord, Who is worthy to be praised, and I am saved from my enemies" (2 Samuel 22:1-4 AMP).

And so, you have to trust that God, Who has begun a good work in you, will perform it unto the day of Jesus Christ. Once you use your faith to slay this giant, you will see him no more. In the past, perhaps you used willpower. Perhaps you tried the ways of man's devices. But this time you will use faith to defeat the enemy, and you won't have to fight this giant again.

It is important to understand that God is the One Who will save you from this enemy who wants to destroy your health. Trust God and relax so that you can accept this new lifestyle as normal. If you don't get to the point of trust, you will receive the blessing, but you will live in such fear that you won't enjoy it. You're not free until you come to the point of *trusting God with the victory.*

Your mind must be renewed to the new level of trusting God to protect your victory. As your body is calibrated to its new size, your mind must adjust to new thinking. God will keep you where you want to be. Encourage yourself by saying, "This is gonna last. It's not going to change. And I don't have to go out there and behead any more fat giants. I'm going to rest in what God has given me the grace to experience. This new lifestyle is going to be normal for me."

You can't spend the rest of your life in bondage to fat grams. You must move on to a level of trust, where you can rest without the anxiety of worrying about your weight. Then you can pursue other adventures, enjoy your career, and raise your children without a preoccupation with food.

Don't give up until your new lifestyle brings freedom. Don't give up faith in becoming the person you want to be until graduation day, when you can exchange your hard work for trust in God's rest.

Carry the Bag of Transferable Truth

I call the five weapons outlined in this book, "The Stones of Transferable Truth." These truths of motivation, understanding, conviction, knowledge, and trust can be used to slay any giant that may threaten to rob you of the abundant life God wants you to enjoy. Let these stones become a part of your personal arsenal against your giants and draw from the bag whenever you need it!

A Note from Carlo

From the creation of man, diet has been a very important part of our lives. Over the years, we have sought and developed new methods of producing and processing food to achieve a higher level of nourishment.

Nutritional information has been modified as more details are discovered about how different substances and micronutrients react to each other and affect the body. These scientific advances help us to understand more clearly how the human body works, and thus enable us to eat a more healthy diet.

Today, due to fast food restaurants and drive-thrus, microwave ovens, and constant advertising, it is easy to eat much more food than the body actually needs. Thus, many people are overweight. Fortunately, science has achieved processes to eliminate or reduce some of the more damaging elements contained in foods, such as fat.

The best way for a person to reduce their weight is to reduce their intake of fat. Some changes in your grocery list will be able to remove those annoying pounds. A diet to lose weight does not need to be monotonous and boring or leave you unsatisfied.

Using Energy

To achieve a successful diet, you must learn how your body operates and how it reacts to various foods. Often we eat foods and have no idea how they will affect our body.

There are three basic food groups: carbohydrates, proteins, and fats. Every person requires all three groups, but the quantities vary from each group depending on the individual. An athlete or someone who engages in regular physical activity will require more calories than a sedentary person.

Other factors to take into account are age, height, and sex. Even though it is certain that reducing fats is a great way to lose weight, this process is limited, because the body will make adjustments. It will convert carbohydrates to fat. Then the amount of carbohydrates will also have to be limited.

To explain this more clearly, our bodies accumulate fats in muscular tissue as well as subcutaneous tissue, where fat is in reserve for the future. If the individual does not use the energy that is accumulated, the body will store more and more fat, and the process is endless.

The only way to use energy in the form of fat and not let it accumulate is through physical exercise. Every movement we make requires energy, which will be taken from the fat storage of the body. The more you exercise, the more fat you will be using.

Say, for example, a person eats 5000 calories a day and uses only 2000. The other 3000 calories are immediately stored. If this process continues, the person will have gained a considerable amount of weight in just two months.

Equivalencies

To establish the energy value of foods for physical activity, science created a measure called the calorie. A calorie is the measure of energy found in each nutrient.

We can calculate how many calories we use in every physical activity.

We can also calculate how much physical activity is necessary to use the calories we have eaten. If we use 1800 to 2000 calories of energy per day, we should not eat more than 1800 to 2000 calories a day.

On the other hand, if we burn 2000 calories a day, but we eat 2200 calories per day, an extra 200 calories are being stored in our body each day. If this continues 15 days, we would gain 1 pound.

3000 stored calories = 1 pound gained

For example, 10 French fries is equal to 200 calories. If you eat 10 French fries a day and the calories are stored instead of burned for six months, you would gain 12 pounds.

Here are some other examples of equivalencies:

Food	Physical Activity
Double hamburger w/cheese - 900 calories	Walk 2 hours (8 miles)
Slice pizza (1/4) - 450 calories	Swim 50 minutes (2 miles)
Chocolate Milkshake - 800 calories	Bicycle 1 hour (14 miles)

Stages of A Diet

1. *Psychological*

Before doing anything, you will have to accept that you have a weight problem and want to solve it. To understand this from the beginning is very important. It is a great help to set a goal — 7 to 10 days, for example — to devote all your energy to the new diet.

A Note from Carlo

Decide from the beginning that you will be different at the end of this time period.

2. *Restrictive*

This stage is difficult because the body is not receiving the food to which it is accustomed. It is also receiving less food while increasing physical activity, and slowly the fat reserves are being used. This process can be accompanied by light headaches and other discomfort as the body adapts to the new diet and regular exercise. At the end of this stage, you may experience some depression.

3. *Adaptation*

You feel like you have a new life, as if you were another person. Everything looks better because you look better. You want to update your wardrobe, and you begin to reevaluate your life. At this point it is important to remember that you have changed your weight and figure, but you must change the mental and emotional causes for being overweight.

4. *Maintenance*

This is the most difficult stage. You must learn to live as the new person you are by continuing the diet. Just because you have reached your desired weight does not mean you can begin eating like you did when you were overweight. You can celebrate from time to time, but not often. To maintain your desired weight, you must maintain the new metabolism by continuing to eat a good, nutritional diet. Remember that life offers many pleasures and rewards besides food!

Tips for Healthy Living

Eat three meals and two snacks every three hours every day.

Eat 70% of your calories by 2:00 in the afternoon.

Eat most of your carbohydrates for lunch.

Eat mostly protein for dinner.

Quit eating by 7:00 at night

Exercise at least four hours a week.

Never do two hard things at the same time.

Never put two bad foods together in the same meal.

A Note from Carlo

Pay the Price

We have to pay a price for the food we choose to eat either by becoming overweight or by burning the calories, through exercise or restrictive intake. The body is a mathematically balanced creation that was designed to equalize its intake of fuel and output of energy.

The good news is that our body is not like a car, which depreciates with use. As you drive a car, the tires wear out, the engine gets worn, and the paint chips off. But the body is designed to become better the more you use it. As you exercise, the body becomes stronger and more beautiful because it is being used.

Do some vigorous exercise you enjoy that gets your heart rate up. All the exercise you do after the first thirty minutes is what will burn off the extra fat. If you think you are too busy, remember you only need to find four hours a week to begin making the change that leads to more enjoyable health and fitness.

There are 168 hours in the week, but your new routine to fitness will only take four hours. Keep the rest of the time for yourself, but give four hours of exercise in dedication to your new life. Remember, these four hours will start making you eat better, feel better, and look better.

Make a Date with Your Ticket to Health

Find a time to exercise that works for you and protect it from other appointments. You can pick the day and time that you want to take your first walk. See how many miles you can walk in that hour. Then you can calculate how many calories you used in that hour. The next day your legs and your feet may be sore, but you have to keep going. Your body appreciates with use. The more you use it, the more it improves. This is the most important date you can make.

Eventually, increase the pace of your walk to be sure you are spending your four hours a week wisely by elevating your heart rate. You need to burn as many calories during this time as you can. Calories make you overweight.

You will lose weight and get in better shape if you start cutting the intake of calories, and then walk to give your body an exhaust system for using the calories that are already in storage. If you take in less and burn more energy you will eventually come to your real weight.

Exercise is so important that even if you keep eating the same food, but you begin walking (or exercising in some manner) for four hours a week, you will burn calories you were not burning before.

Only exercising will help, but the time it will take you to lose weight is going to be less if you also restrict your intake of calories and fat. If the change is too slow, you may become discouraged and give up.

Don't Be Tempted by Quick Weight-Loss Programs

Fast diets are not safe or healthy. You will, however, see quick results if you combine four hours of exercise each week and restrict your intake of calories and fat grams. You will feel the change in the way your body moves and acts. Your clothes will fit differently. In fact, you will feel so much better, it will be difficult for you to give up this better way of life once you experience it.

A Note from Carlo

If your doctor has told you to eat 1400 calories per day while you are losing weight, you can have good food during this restrictive time of your diet.

- Your breakfast should be 400 calories
- You should eat a carbohydrate snack of about 150 calories about two or three hours after breakfast.
- Eat a lunch of 400 calories before 2:00 PM.
- Eat another snack of 150 calories within 1 to 3 hours.
- Eat a 300-calorie dinner before 6:30 PM.

Snacks can be any fat-free food or a fruit such as a banana, pear, apple, etc. Always get low-calorie products during this restrictive phase of eating. There are fat-free breads, soft drinks, jams, cookies, and dressings. Make your kitchen user-friendly by clearing out the old foods and filling it with nonfat alternatives.

Here is a sample of what you could have in three meals and 2 snacks:

Breakfast:	Cereal with skim milk and a banana.
	Two fat-free eggs with a slice of fat-free ham.
Morning snack:	Any snack with carbohydrates.
Lunch:	Any pasta with green salad and fat-free dressing.
Afternoon snack:	Apple and fat-free pudding.
Dinner:	Chicken breast with any kind of salad or green vegetables.

If at any time you feel dizzy, stop what you are doing and eat something, even if you break your diet.

I realize that the above menu could be more food than you are presently eating. The difference is, finding fat-free alternatives during this time of losing weight. Later you will be able to increase the fat grams again, when you are maintaining your real body weight.

Choose Foods That Will Build Your Strength

When possible, use fresh vegetables and juices. Frozen foods are almost as good as the fresh, but it is better to use fresh when possible. When you have to travel or be away from home, take a healthy snack with you or go to the supermarket and buy a couple of things that will keep you from being hungry, but are still good for you.

You can take a sandwich of lean ham and fat-free cheese with crunchy vegetables, such as celery or cucumbers. Soybean is one of the best proteins for us to eat. There are some vegie-burgers at the supermarket made of soybean, gluten, mushrooms, and spices, which have an excellent flavor. Microwave one and put it on a bun with lettuce and mustard, and you will have a delicious meal or snack.

Always carry a couple of snacks with you so you won't get hungry. It isn't good to go too long without food. Keeping a snack with a hundred to two hundred calories close at hand is excellent during this time of cutting back calories. This will keep you in control of your appetite. If you get too hungry, you might be tempted to eat foods you shouldn't.

Increase Your Self-control

Fasting is one of the ways to strengthen your power to get to your goal. It is excellent if you can go twelve to thirty-six hours without food for one or two days each month. It is easier to do this when you are convinced it is something that is going to help you. You will soon see that you have better skin, better digestion, and a better disposition. When you get used to fasting, you will become sensitive to knowing when your body needs a fast.

On the day you fast, drink as much water as you can. Drink decaf fruit teas and juices. The best are pineapple, grapefruit, and oranges. Be sure you are drinking only the juice. Don't put these fruits in a blender, because then you are actually eating fruits. Use a juicer and throw away the pulp on the day you are drinking only liquids. Look for the juices that are 100 percent fruit juice.

Even children have days when they say, "I don't want to eat." Their bodies are asking for a break. It's very healthy to let our systems relax and refresh. Even the animals do things to help themselves. I have seen many dogs eat grass because they instinctively know they need it.

Many times we know our body has had too much food. Fasting may be hard the first time, but it is after we do the right thing that the reward comes. You will feel better, and your body is going to be better because it really needs a break.

When you are fasting, you shouldn't try to also do a strenuous workout. If you have an important meeting on the day you normally fast, then pick another day to fast. Never do two hard things at the same time. You will be more successful if you always balance your activities as well as your foods.

It is difficult to give up something you want, but it increases your willpower to practice resisting things that are not good for you. This practice will strengthen your resistance to other temptations besides food.

I know some people who take cold showers even if it's cold outside, because the cold water stimulates the blood stream and enhances their circulation. The first time I did this, it was very hard for me!

We believe we should not spoil our bodies. Your body can do more than you think. The more you pamper your body, the weaker your body becomes. You know that it isn't good to spoil a child. The same is true of your own body. You shouldn't overprotect it to the point of making it too lazy. Work is better for your body than idleness.

Decrease Your Worries

To be thin and in shape is not a key to happiness, but at least good health is something you don't have to worry about. If you find a solution to being healthy, you are able to think about something else. It is good not to have to worry about your health.

These guidelines are not a key for happiness, but they are the key for taking off the weight so you don't have to worry about that burden anymore. You will feel like someone took weight off of your shoulders when the doctor tells you "Don't worry about your health. You are one hundred percent healthy right now."

We don't have to be thin to be happy, but poor health certainly can keep us from happiness.

It is important to have knowledge and understanding of how to eat right. You are never too old to enjoy activity and good health. When you understand the basic requirements of exercise and nutrition, they become a part of your conscience.

Understanding will cause you to make good decisions without hesitating. And the knowledge of what is good for you and what isn't is something you learn a little bit at a time. But if you understand why certain foods are not as healthy for you and how your body works, you will be able to use common sense to make good choices.

Good health is a reflection of good lifestyle choices. And yes, the reward of a good lifestyle is happiness.

Maintain Your Goal

Many people reach their real weight within three months of cutting calories and exercising at least four hours a week. Once you are your ideal weight, your body may fight to put on the cloak of fat again, thinking that it needs it to survive.

You will need to keep focused on your new lifestyle of healthy eating and exercise for six months after your weight is gone. In that time, your body will adapt to the new weight and will be convinced that you do not need the storage supply of extra energy.

Once your body has maintained your new weight for six months, you will be able to increase your calories, maintain your exercise program, and enjoy a good life, free from the burden of extra weight.

Basic Recipes

What follows are some of the recipes I have created for people like Bishop Jakes, who desire to lose weight and get their bodies in good physical shape. However, every person is different, and what is good for one person may not be good for another. To specify a diet and exercise plan just for you, please contact me at cgabrelian@aol.com.

Sauce Fifth Avenue

We have created a combination of special ingredients to season food — fat-free — and we call it Sauce Fifth Avenue. Fat-free food can have flavor! This sauce can be prepared in large quantities and kept in a bottle for daily use. It does not need to be refrigerated, and it is very easy to make.

2 cups soy sauce
1 cup Worcestershire sauce
1 cup white wine

1 teaspoon pepper
2 teaspoons brown sugar
1 pinch salt

Combination of Herbs for Seasoning

In general, I do not use salt and pepper in cooking. It is best to stay away from salt, especially to maintain good health. If you must, use a little salt and pepper to taste. **In all my recipes that call for "herbs," I am referring to the following "Combination of Herbs for Seasoning."** This recipe can be done in greater quantities since it is in continuous use.

1 1/2 cup dried basil
1 cup thyme
1 cup dried oregano

2 teaspoons pepper
1/4 cup sage

All these ingredients are ground or mashed. Once combined, the seasoning can be kept in a bottle for daily use. It does not require refrigeration.

Breakfast

Corn Pancakes

8 pancakes

Per Serving

Calories 150
Fat grams 1

1/2 cup all-purpose flour
1 teaspoon baking powder
1 teaspoon sugar
1/2 cup cornmeal
1 egg white
1 cup fat-free milk
1/2 cup applesauce
Nonfat, nonstick spray

Combine in a bowl flour, baking powder, sugar, and cornmeal. In another bowl mix egg white, milk, and applesauce. Fold into flour mixture. Spray baking dish with nonfat, nonstick spray and pour pancakes. Bake at 350° for 12 to 15 minutes.

Waffles with Sausage

6 plums
4 envelopes noncaloric sugar substitute
4 cups waffle flour
1 cup fat-free eggs
2 cups fat-free milk
2 teaspoons fat-free butter
Nonfat, nonstick spray
2 fat-free sausages

Serves 4

Per Serving
Calories 310
Fat grams 1

Remove seeds from plums and boil in a little water. When they are tender, add noncaloric sugar substitute and mash into paste. Set aside. Combine flour, eggs, milk, and butter in blender and beat well. Slice sausage into strips and sauté until browned. Spray waffle iron with nonfat, nonstick spray and add mixture. When waffles are done, serve with a little fat-free butter, plum sauce, and sausage strips.

Spanish Omelet

Serves 4

Per Serving

Calories   180
Fat grams   2

Nonfat, nonstick spray
1 teaspoon minced garlic
1/2 cup pearl onions
1/2 cup green pepper
1 cup peas
1 cup spaghetti sauce
1/2 pound fat-free sausage
2 cups egg beaters

Spray skillet with nonfat, nonstick spray and sauté garlic, onions, and green pepper. Add peas and spaghetti sauce. Set aside. Cook on low heat 5 minutes. In a separate skillet, sauté sausage. In another skillet, make omelet, putting sausage in the middle before folding over. Top with sauce and serve.

French Toast with Peaches

Serves 4

Per Serving

Calories   205
Fat grams   1

1 sliced peach
1 teaspoon lemon juice
3 envelopes noncaloric sugar substitute
1/2 teaspoon cinnamon
1/2 teaspoon nutmeg
Nonfat, nonstick spray
8 low-fat bread slices
1 cup egg beaters
1 cup honey or low-calorie maple syrup

Cook peaches with a little water, lemon juice, noncaloric sugar substitute, cinnamon, and nutmeg until tender. Spray skillet with nonfat, nonstick spray and heat. Dip bread slices in egg and place in skillet. Turn. When done, serve at once with honey or syrup and peaches.

Strawberry Crepes

16 sliced strawberries
8 envelopes noncaloric sugar substitute
8 cups fat-free milk
3 teaspoons cornstarch
1 teaspoon vanilla
4 cups pancake flour
1/2 cup egg beaters

Serves 4

Per Serving
Calories   375
Fat grams   2

Jam:
Boil strawberries with a little water. When tender add 4 envelopes noncaloric sugar substitute and stir over low heat for 15 minutes.

Pudding:
Warm 4 milk cups in microwave and stir in (preferably with plastic spoon) the following in small amounts, heating mixture in microwave for 30 seconds each time an amount is added: cornstarch mixed with 1/2 cup cold water, 4 envelopes noncaloric sugar substitute, and vanilla. Do this until thickened.

Crepe:
In a blender, mix flour, egg, and 4 cups milk. Cook crepe like a pancake, but it will be very thin, and fill with pudding. Serve hot with jam on top.

Banana Pancakes

Serves 12

Per Serving

Calories   220
Fat grams   3

1 banana
1 teaspoon vanilla
1/2 cup orange juice
1 cup sugar
1/2 cup all-purpose flour
1/2 cup coconut
1 teaspoon baking powder
1/2 teaspoon salt
4 egg whites, beaten until stiff
1/2 cup dried fruit

Puree banana, vanilla, and orange juice. Sift sugar, flour, coconut, baking powder, and salt in a bowl. Stir in banana mixture, egg whites, and dried fruit. Pour into pan and bake at 350° for 35 minutes.

Strawberry Omelet with Banana

Serves 4

Per Serving

Calories   180
Fat grams   1

2 cups sliced strawberries
1 sliced banana
3 teaspoons lemon juice
4 envelopes noncaloric sugar substitute
Nonfat, nonstick spray
8 slices fat-free bacon
2 cups egg beaters

In a bowl combine strawberries, banana, lemon juice and noncaloric sugar substitute. Set aside. Spray skillet with nonfat, nonstick spray and sauté bacon. Set aside. Spray skillet with nonfat, nonstick spray and cook egg. Before folding omelet, fill with strawberry mixture. Serve with bacon.

Ham Biscuits

4 cups fat-free pancake flour
1 cup fat-free egg
1 cup fat-free milk
1 apple, sliced
4 envelopes noncaloric sugar substitute
1 teaspoon cinnamon
1 teaspoon nutmeg
1/2 pound fat-free ham, sliced
8 slices fat-free American cheese
4 slices melon

Serves 4

Per Serving
Calories   380
Fat grams   1

Mix flour with egg and milk, beating until very thick. Form into golf ball size balls. Press balls flat and bake 20 minutes at 350°. On low heat, boil apple slices in a little water with noncaloric sugar substitute, cinnamon, and nutmeg. Cut biscuits in half and put a slice of ham, teaspoon of apple mixture, and slice of cheese in middle. Garnish with a slice of melon.

Soda Bread

2 cups wheat flour
1 cup all-purpose flour
1 teaspoon baking powder
1 teaspoon baking soda
1 1/2 fat-free buttermilk
Nonfat, nonstick spray

Serves 9

Per Serving
Calories   125
Fat grams   0

Combine in a bowl flour, baking powder, and baking soda. Add buttermilk. Beat vigorously 2 minutes and form into small balls. Put balls on baking sheet sprayed with nonfat, nonstick spray. Bake at 350° for 30 minutes.

Salads

Potato Salad

Serves 4

Per Serving

Calories 130
Fat grams 0

4 boiled Idaho potatoes, cubed
3 boiled eggs, diced
4 teaspoons sweet pickle relish
1 cup diced celery
1/2 cup diced white onion
1 cup diced cucumber
2 teaspoons brown sugar
5 teaspoons fat-free mayonnaise
2 teaspoons fat-free ranch dressing
3 teaspoons mustard

Mix all the ingredients in a bowl.

Salad Jimena

Serves 4

Per Serving

Calories 92
Fat grams 0

1 head romaine lettuce, sliced
2 sliced boiled eggs
1 sliced tomato
1/2 sliced red pepper
4 slices fat-free ham
4 slices fat-free American cheese cut in strips
4 slices fat-free turkey breast cut in strips
4 strawberries
Fat-free seasoning

Put the sliced lettuce in a bowl and adorn with others ingredients. Use fat-free seasoning.

Chicken Salad with Beans

3 chicken breasts, without skin
salt and pepper
1 chopped head iceberg lettuce
2 cups cooked green beans
2 cups fresh sliced mushrooms
2 cups cherry tomatoes cut in halves
2 teaspoons herbs
2 teaspoons honey
2 teaspoons mustard
2 teaspoons vinegar
2 teaspoons lemon juice
1 teaspoon chopped chives
1/2 melon, sliced

Serves 4

Per Serving
Calories   250
Fat grams   2

Roast chicken in oven with salt and pepper. Cut in cubes. In salad bowl, put lettuce, chicken, beans, mushrooms, and tomatoes. Sprinkle with herbs. Dressing: Combine honey and mustard and beat vigorously. Add vinegar, lemon juice, and chives. Pour on salad. Serve melon on the side.

Salad Veronica

2 cups diced celery
2 cups chopped red apple
2 cups chopped pineapple in water
2 cups fat-free yogurt
1/2 cup raisins
2 teaspoons chopped nuts

Serves 4

Per Serving
Calories   200
Fat grams   4

Combine first five ingredients and top with nuts.

Farfale Salad with Ham

Serves 4

Per Serving

Calories 325
Fat grams 3

1 bag farfale noodles
3 small onions, cut in strips
1 sliced red pepper
1 sliced green pepper
1 sliced yellow pepper
1 pound fat-free ham in 1/2-inch cubes
1/2 head Romaine lettuce, sliced
1/2 cup black olives, without pits and cut in half
1 teaspoon herbs
1 cup fat-free Italian seasoning

Cook noodles, rinsing immediately with cold water. Sauté onion and peppers. Combine all ingredients in a bowl with seasonings. Serve cold if you prefer, topped with fat-free parmesan cheese.

Stuffed Tomatoes with Tuna

Serves 4

Per Serving

Calories 90
Fat grams 0

1 large can tuna in water
1/2 cup chopped onion
2 boiled egg whites, chopped
1/2 cup chopped lettuce
1/2 cup chopped carrot
5 teaspoons fat-free mayonnaise
2 teaspoons lime juice
4 leaves romaine lettuce
4 tomatoes

Combine all ingredients except lettuce and tomatoes. Place each tomato on a leaf of lettuce. Make a hole in the tomatoes and fill with the mixture of all the other ingredients.

Shrimp Salad

8 cups shrimp
1 cup Sauce Fifth Avenue
1 cup lemon juice
1 teaspoon mustard
3 teaspoons herbs
4 heads Boston lettuce
4 slices avocado
4 slices cucumber
8 cherry tomatoes

Serves 4

Per Serving
Calories   200
Fat grams   3

Marinate shrimp in Sauce Fifth Avenue, lemon juice, mustard, and herbs at least 2 hours. Put mixture into lettuce leaves and garnish with avocado, cucumber, and tomatoes. Refrigerate 10 minutes before serving.

Salad Treviso

1/2 pound fat-free Philadelphia cream cheese
1/2 teaspoon garlic powder
1 teaspoon white vinegar
4 teaspoons fresh basil
2 sliced red tomatoes
2 sliced yellow tomatoes

Serves 4

Per Serving
Calories   130
Fat grams   0

Blend cheese with garlic, vinegar, and half of the fresh basil into a sauce. Put tomatoes on plate top with sauce. Garnish with remaining basil.

Vegetables

Risotto Primavera

Serves 4

Per Serving
Calories   185
Fat grams   0

2 cups rice
1 package vegetables with broccoli, carrots, mushrooms, and cauliflower
1 sliced red pepper
1 sliced green pepper
1 teaspoon herbs
3 teaspoons fat-free butter

Cook rice. Steam vegetables (including red and green pepper) and mix with herbs and butter. In a large bowl mix vegetables with rice. Serve with salt and pepper and a little butter.

New Potatoes

Serves 4

Per Serving
Calories   130
Fat grams   0

1 pound red potatoes, cut in halves
2 teaspoons rosemary
1 teaspoon herbs
1 teaspoon minced garlic
Nonfat, nonstick spray
1 sprig parsley
2 teaspoons paprika

Combine first four ingredients in a bowl. Spray baking dish with nonfat, nonstick spray, pour mixture into it, and cover with aluminum foil. Bake at 350° until potatoes are cooked. Serve garnished with parsley and paprika.

Zucchini with Corn

Nonfat, nonstick spray
1/2 chopped onion
1 green pepper, thinly sliced
8 zucchini, cubed
2 cups yellow corn
2 teaspoons herbs
1 diced tomato
2 teaspoons Sauce Fifth Avenue
1/2 cup fat-free cream
8 corn tortillas

Serves 4

Per Serving
Calories   250
Fat grams   2

Spray skillet with nonfat, nonstick spray and sauté onion and green pepper until tender. Add other ingredients except tortillas, cover, and bring to boil. Serve with tortillas and a little cream.

Beans with Sausage

Nonfat, nonstick spray
3 teaspoons chopped onion
2 teaspoons minced garlic
4 cups beans
2 teaspoons herbs
1 fat-free kielbasa sausage, cut in strips
4 teaspoons fat-free butter

Serves 4

Per Serving
Calories   250
Fat grams   0

Spray skillet with nonfat, nonstick spray and sauté onion with garlic. Add beans and herbs. Then add sausage and fat-free butter.

Moros and Christian

Serves 4

Per Serving

Calories   275
Fat grams   2

3 cups black beans
1 onion
1 clove garlic
2 cups cooked rice
2 teaspoons herbs
1 green pepper
1 tomato
1 sprig parsley
1 bag fat-free corn fritters

Cook beans with 1/2 onion and garlic. Cook and drain rice. Drain beans and mix with rice in a bowl with herbs. Steep green pepper, tomato, and remaining onion for pico de gallo sauce. Serve beans and rice hot with 2 teaspoons sauce on top, garnished with parsley and fritters on the side.

Corn and Red Pepper

Serves 4

Per Serving

Calories   70
Fat grams   1

1 teaspoon minced garlic
2 teaspoons chopped scallion
4 cups yellow sweet corn
1 cup finely chopped red pepper
1 teaspoon herbs
3 teaspoons Sauce Fifth Avenue
1/2 teaspoon brown sugar
3 teaspoons fat-free butter

Sauté garlic and scallion. Add corn, red pepper, and herbs and cook on low heat 5 minutes. Add Sauce Fifth Avenue, brown sugar, and butter. Salt and pepper to taste.

Peas with Pearl Onions

4 cups peas
2 cups pearl onions
2 teaspoons herbs
6 teaspoons fat-free butter
1 cup fat-free cream
4 teaspoons bread crumbs
1 sprig fresh parsley

Serves 4

Per Serving
Calories   130
Fat grams   0

Preheat oven to 350°. Combine first six ingredients and bake 20 minutes. Adorn with parsley.

Spinach with Bacon

Nonfat, nonstick spray
1/2 pound finely chopped fat-free bacon
4 teaspoons minced garlic
2 pounds stemless spinach
1/2 cup Sauce Fifth Avenue
4 slices tomato

Serves 4

Per Serving
Calories   90
Fat grams   0

Spray skillet with nonfat, nonstick spray. Sauté bacon and garlic. Add spinach. When spinach is cooked add Sauce Fifth Avenue. Garnish with tomato.

Aztec Potato

Nonfat, nonstick spray
2 pounds boiled sliced potatoes
2 cups fat-free cream
10 slices fat-free ham
10 slices low-fat cheese

Serves 4

Per Serving
Calories   430
Fat grams   0

Spray casserole dish with nonfat, nonstick spray. Layer potatoes, cream, ham, and cheese. Repeat until all ingredients are gone. Cover pan with aluminum foil and bake at 350° for 20 minutes.

Rice with Lentils

Serves 4

Per Serving

Calories 287
Fat grams 4

4 cups rice
4 cups lentils
1/2 onion, diced
2 teaspoons minced garlic
2 teaspoons herbs
4 teaspoons chopped fat-free bacon
2 boiled eggs, sliced
4 red pepper slices

Cook rice. Cook lentils, onion, and garlic together in water. Drain and combine with rice in a bowl. Add herbs and bacon. Garnish with egg and red pepper.

Cream of Carrots

Serves 4

Per Serving

Calories 240
Fat grams 1

1 pound carrots, sliced
4 cups fat-free milk
1 cup fat-free cream
8 ounces fat-free cream cheese
1 cup fat-free chicken broth
2 teaspoons herbs
2 toasted low-fat bread slices, cut into croutons

Cook carrots with a little water until tender. Drain and combine with remaining ingredients except croutons. Cook on low heat 15 minutes. Garnish with croutons.

Potatoes with Green Pepper

4 Idaho potatoes, cubed
1 teaspoon herbs
Nonfat, nonstick spray
1 onion in one-inch squares
2 green peppers in one-inch squares
Fat-free butter

Serves 4

Per Serving
Calories   120
Fat grams   0

Boil potatoes with herbs until almost ready. Rinse them with cold water and drain. Spray skillet with nonfat, nonstick spray and sauté onion and green pepper. When cooked, add potatoes. When potatoes are cooked, you can put a little fat-free butter on them and serve.

Celery with Cream Cheese and Raisins

Serves 4

1 cup fat-free Philadelphia cream cheese
1/2 cup raisins
3 teaspoons low calorie peach jam
4 celery stalks, cut in chunks
1 sliced peach

Per Serving
Calories   160
Fat grams   1

Combine cheese, raisins, and jam. Fill celery with the paste and serve with peach slices.

Soups

Lentil Soup

Serves 4

2 cups lentils
Nonfat, nonstick spray
2 teaspoons minced garlic
1/2 cup chopped onion
1 cup chopped carrots
1 cup tomato paste
1 cup chopped potatoes
1 cup fat-free chicken broth
1/2 pound ham, cubed
1 sliced plantain

Per Serving

Calories   300
Fat grams   3

Boil lentils in water until half cooked. In sprayed skillet, sauté garlic and onion. Add carrots and tomato paste. Combine all ingredients except plantain into pot and cook on low heat until done. Add plantain a few minutes before serving.

Scallop Soup

Serves 4

Nonfat, nonstick spray
2 pounds scallops
1 cup small onions cut in strips
2 cups tomatoes, mashed
4 teaspoons minced garlic
2 teaspoons Sauce Fifth Avenue
2 teaspoons herbs
1 cup water

Per Serving

Calories   250
Fat grams   2

Spray skillet with nonfat, nonstick spray. Sauté scallops, onion, and garlic 10 minutes. Add Sauce Fifth Avenue. When scallops are dark red, add remaining ingredients and cook 20 minutes on low heat.

Tomato Soup

2 1/2 pounds tomatoes
1 tablespoon fat-free butter
4 scallions, chopped
4 cloves garlic, minced
2 1/2 cups fat-free chicken broth
4 tablespoons fresh basil, minced
1 bay leaf
2 teaspoons sugar
1/2 cup white wine
2 cups tomatoes, chopped
1 tablespoon parsley, minced

Serves 6

Per Serving

Calories	187
Fat grams	1

Place tomatoes in boiling water for about 30 seconds. Remove and peel skins. Quarter and remove seeds, then puree in blender 1 minute. Heat butter in saucepan and sauté chopped scallions until transparent. Add garlic and tomatoes. Lower heat and simmer 5 minutes. Stir in chicken broth, herbs, and sugar. Cover and simmer 30 minutes. Add wine and chopped tomatoes and cook another 15 minutes. Remove from heat and stir in parsley.

Potato and Leeks Soup

Serves 4

5 cups potatoes, cut in strips
Nonfat, nonstick spray
2 cups leeks, cut in strips
2 teaspoons minced garlic
1 cup tomato paste
4 cups fat-free chicken broth

Per Serving

Calories	160
Fat grams	0

Precook potatoes and drain. Spray pan with nonfat, nonstick spray and sauté leeks and garlic. When leeks are cooked, add tomato paste, potatoes, and broth. Simmer on low heat until hot.

Chicken Soup Venezia

Serves 4

Per Serving

Calories 175
Fat grams 0

4 chicken breasts, without bone or skin
salt and pepper to taste
1 teaspoon garlic powder
Nonfat, nonstick spray
2 stalks broccoli, cut in pieces
4 small onions, diced
1 red pepper, diced
1 cup baby carrots, cut in pieces
6 cups water
2 teaspoons fat-free chicken broth
1 sprig parsley

Roast chicken with salt, pepper, and garlic. Cut in cubes. Spray large saucepan with nonfat, nonstick spray and add vegetables. Sauté. Add water, broth, and chicken. Salt and pepper to taste. Boil 15 minutes on low heat. Serve soup topped with parsley.

Soup Virginia

Serves 4

Per Serving

Calories 60
Fat grams 0

1/2 onion, diced
2 teaspoons minced garlic
2 cups diced carrots
2 cups chopped celery
2 cups diced zucchini
2 cups diced squash
2 cups diced mushrooms
3 cups tomato sauce
4 teaspoons herbs
4 teaspoons Sauce Fifth Avenue
4 cups water

Spray pan with nonfat, nonstick spray. Sauté onion, garlic, carrots, and celery 10 minutes. Add zucchini, squash, and mushrooms and fry 10 minutes. Add remaining ingredients except water and cook 5 minutes. Add water and cook on low heat 10 minutes. Ready to be served.

Spinach Soup

1 cup water
1 release leek
1 carrot, peeled and sliced
1 celery stalk, sliced
6 cups fat-free chicken broth
6 release bunches fresh spinach, stems removed
3 tablespoons fat-free parmesan cheese, freshly grated

Serves 8

Per Serving
Calories   150
Fat grams   0

Bring to boil water, leek, carrot, and celery. Reduce heat and simmer until vegetables are tender. Add chicken broth and bring to boil. Add spinach and cook 2 minutes uncovered, until spinach wilts. Transfer to food processor in small batches. Puree until very smooth. Transfer to large pot. This soup will change color if left standing, so serve immediately, garnished with grated cheese.

Meat, Chicken, & Fish

Ham and Melon

Serves 4

Per Serving

Calories   300
Fat grams   1

1/2 cup mustard
1 teaspoon lemon juice
2 teaspoons honey
1 teaspoon mint
1 cantaloupe, in balls
1 pound fat-free smoked ham, thickly sliced squares
1 honeydew melon, in balls

Puree mustard with lemon, honey, and mint in blender. On a skewer string a ball of cantaloupe, a strip of ham and a ball of honeydew. Serve with mustard sauce.

Liver and Onions

Serves 4

Per Serving

Calories   310
Fat grams   4

4 liver filets
1/2 cup white wine
3 teaspoons herbs
1 teaspoon garlic powder
Nonfat, nonstick spray
2 sliced onions
1 cup all-purpose flour

Marinate liver in wine, herbs, and garlic powder 2 hours. Caramelize onions and remove from heat. Coat liver with flour. Spray skillet with nonfat, nonstick spray and add liver. Fry on high heat until done. Serve with onion.

Sausage with Potatoes

4 potatoes, cubed
2 large tomatoes
1/2 onion, sliced
1 clove garlic
2 teaspoons herbs
3 cups water
1 1/2 pounds fat-free sausages
1 bag fat-free corn fritters

Serves 4

Per Serving
Calories   325
Fat grams   1

Cook potatoes until almost tender. Puree tomatoes, onion, garlic, herbs, and water. Sauté 10 minutes. Add potatoes and sausages, cut in strips. Serve garnished with corn fritters.

Chicken Parmesan

4 beaten chicken breasts, without skin
2 teaspoons Sauce Fifth Avenue
2 teaspoons herbs
1 teaspoon garlic powder
2 cups bread crumbs
1/2 cup fat-free parmesan cheese
Nonfat, nonstick spray

Serves 4

Per Serving
Calories   180
Fat grams   2

Marinate chicken in Sauce Fifth Avenue, herbs, and garlic powder. In a bowl mix bread crumbs and cheese. Bread chicken breasts with bread crumb and cheese mixture. Spray skillet with nonfat, nonstick spray and sauté chicken until done and brown on both sides. Can be served with pasta.

Chicken Rosemary

Serves 4

1 entire chicken
4 teaspoons herbs
3 teaspoons garlic powder
4 teaspoons rosemary

Per Serving

Calories   200
Fat grams   4

Season chicken with all ingredients and bake 1 hour, 15 minutes at 300°. Just before serving, brown 5 minutes. May garnish with bed of lettuce or vegetables.

Chicken Rolls

Serves 4

4 beaten chicken breasts, without bone or skin
2 teaspoons herbs
4 teaspoons Sauce Fifth Avenue
2 teaspoons garlic powder
4 slices fat-free ham
toothpicks
Nonfat, nonstick spray

Per Serving

Calories   250
Fat grams   2

Marinate chicken with herbs, Sauce Fifth Avenue, and garlic powder for 2 hours. Take a chicken breast and a slice of ham and roll together. Insert toothpick to hold. Spray skillet with nonfat, nonstick spray and sauté rolls until dark red color.

Chicken and Rice

Nonfat, nonstick cooking spray
1 pound chicken breasts, without bone or skin, cut into pieces
2 teaspoons fat-free butter
1 release onion, chopped
2 cloves garlic, minced
2 1/2 cups defatted chicken broth
1/4 cup sherry vinegar
1 release green pepper, seeded, diced
1 release red pepper, seeded, diced
1/2 teaspoon ground saffron
1/2 teaspoon black pepper
1/2 teaspoon cayenne pepper
1 1/2 cups uncooked long grain white rice
1 1/2 cups green peas (fresh or frozen)

Serves 7

Per Serving

Calories	275
Fat grams	2

Coat Dutch oven or soup pot with cooking spray. Cook chicken over medium heat, turning frequently, for 6 to 8 minutes or until brown and cooked through. Remove and set aside in mixing bowl. In pot combine oil, onion, garlic, and 3 tablespoons broth. Stir up any brown bits from bottom of pot. Cook over medium heat stirring frequently, 6 or 7 minutes or until onion is tender. Add more broth if too much evaporates. Add remaining broth along with sherry, green pepper, and red pepper. Add chicken. Stir in saffron, black pepper, cayenne pepper, rice, and peas. Bring to boil. Reduce heat and simmer 20 minutes or until rice is tender. Stir before serving.

Chicken Breasts Marsala

Serves 4

2 teaspoons minced garlic
1 cup onion, diced
6 cups sliced mushrooms
Nonfat, nonstick spray
4 slightly beaten chicken breasts
6 teaspoons Sauce Fifth Avenue
2 teaspoons herbs
1 cup Marsala wine
1 cup fat-free chicken broth

Per Serving
Calories   280
Fat grams   1

Sauté garlic and onion until caramelized. Add mushrooms and turn heat off. Spray skillet with nonfat, nonstick spray and sauté chicken breasts with Sauce Fifth Avenue until chicken is a red color. Add herbs and wine. Add mushroom mixture and broth. Simmer 5 minutes.

Shrimp Cocktail

Serves 4

1 pound cooked shrimp (12-16), shelled and deveined
2 teaspoons Sauce Fifth Avenue
2 teaspoons herbs
1/2 cup lemon juice
2 cups catsup
4 slices avocado
2 teaspoons diced onion
8 fat-free soda crackers

Per Serving
Calories   165
Fat grams   2

Marinate shrimp in Sauce Fifth Avenue with herbs and lemon juice at least 2 hours. Add catsup. Serve garnished with avocado, onion, and 2 crackers.

Orange Roughy

4 orange roughy filets
2 teaspoons herbs
4 teaspoons Sauce Fifth Avenue
2 teaspoons lemon juice
1 teaspoon mustard
Nonfat, nonstick spray
4 small onions, cut in strips
1 pound cooked shrimp, shelled and deveined
2 teaspoons minced garlic
1/2 teaspoon tarragon sauce
1 cup tomato paste

Serves 4

Per Serving
Calories   275
Fat grams   2

Marinate filets with herbs, Sauce Fifth Avenue, lemon juice, and mustard. Spray skillet with non-fat, nonstick spray and sauté onions, shrimp, and garlic. Add white wine and tomato paste. Remove shrimp mixture and in the same skillet fry orange roughy filets on low heat until they are a dark red color. Serve topped with shrimp and with rice on the side.

Tuna with Herbs

4 filets tuna
4 teaspoons herbs
2 teaspoons Sauce Fifth Avenue
2 teaspoons garlic powder

Serves 4

Per Serving
Calories   300
Fat grams   4.5

Marinate tuna with all ingredients for 2 hours. Grill. Be careful not to overcook, so tuna does not fall apart.

Fish Rolls

Serves 4

Per Serving

Calories   185
Fat grams   2

4 fresh white fish filets
2 teaspoons herbs
2 teaspoons garlic powder
2 teaspoons Sauce Fifth Avenue
2 teaspoons lemon juice
1/2 teaspoon chopped mint
1/2 teaspoon tarragon sauce
Nonfat, nonstick spray
2 cups sliced mushrooms
1 large tomato, diced
1/2 cup chopped celery
1/2 chopped onion
16 asparagus stalks
toothpicks

Marinate filets with herbs, garlic powder, Sauce Fifth Avenue, lemon juice, mint, and wine. Spray skillet with nonfat, nonstick spray and sauté mushrooms, tomato, celery, and onion. Set topping aside. Remove from heat when tender. Shave asparagus stems down to tender area and boil in water until tender. Roll asparagus in fish filets and fasten with a toothpick. In another sprayed skillet, sauté fish rolls on low heat, covered. Serve covered with topping.

Stuffed Salmon with Shrimp

1 entire salmon
6 teaspoons herbs
4 teaspoons garlic powder
4 teaspoons chopped bay leaf
1/2 cup walnuts
1 pound fat-free Philadelphia cream cheese
3 pounds shrimp for salad
Cherry tomatoes
Baby Carrots
Broccoli, in small pieces
Cauliflower, in small pieces

Serves 10

Per Serving

Calories	300
Fat grams	6

Open salmon like a butterfly and draw out all thorns. Season with herbs, garlic, and bay leaf. If possible, let stand for 2 to 3 hours. Mash nuts and Philadelphia cream cheese into a paste. Stir in shrimp and stuff salmon. Cover with aluminum foil and bake 1 hour at 300°. To serve, garnish with cherry tomatoes, baby carrots, broccoli, and cauliflower.

Scallops Shishkabob

Serves 4

Per Serving
Calories   175
Fat grams   1

1 pound scallops
2 teaspoons herbs
2 teaspoons Sauce Fifth Avenue
1 teaspoon onion powder
2 teaspoons garlic powder
3 teaspoons lemon juice
1 red pepper, cut in squares
1 green pepper, cut in squares
2 squash, cut in squares

Marinate scallops with herbs, Sauce Fifth Avenue, onion powder, garlic powder, and lemon juice. String on skewers, alternating chunks of scallops and vegetables. Cook over grill or in oven until done.

Green Peppers Stuffed with Tuna

Serves 4

Per Serving
Calories   190
Fat grams   1

2 cups tuna in water, drained
1 can peas, drained
1/2 cup fat-free mayonnaise
2 teaspoons vinegar
1 teaspoon rice vinegar
4 green peppers
8 onion rings, roasted
8 cherry tomatoes
1 cup salsa

Combine in a bowl tuna, peas, mayonnaise, vinegar, and wine. Roast green peppers and place them in a plastic bag to sweat 10 minutes. Remove from bag and remove skin and seeds. Fill with tuna mixture. Serve garnished with onion rings, tomatoes, and salsa.

Sandwiches & Pizza

TNU3 Sandwich

8 low-calorie bread slices
4 fat-free cheese slices
8 slices fat-free ham
4 teaspoons fat-free mayonnaise
4 slices avocado
4 slices onion
4 slices green pepper
4 slices tomato
1 package alfalfa sprouts
Mustard

Serves 4

Per Serving
Calories   275
Fat grams   5

Toast bread. Make sandwich with one cheese slice in the middle of 2 slices ham. Add remaining ingredients.

Ham and Cheese Pitas

1/2 pound fat-free ham, sliced
Nonfat, nonstick spray
1 cup onion, sliced
2 cups okra
4 cups mushrooms
2 teaspoons Sauce Fifth Avenue
4 fat-free pita pouches
1 pound fat-free cheese, sliced

Serves 4

Per Serving
Calories   400
Fat grams   0

Warm ham. Spray skillet with nonfat, nonstick spray and sauté onion with okra. Add mushrooms and Sauce Fifth Avenue. Warm bread. Cut one side of bread and put stuffing inside. Put ham in bread. Add cheese. Warm in oven until cheese melts.

Chili Hot Dog

Serves 4

Per Serving

Calories   380
Fat grams   2

4 fat-free hot dogs
4 hot dog buns
1/2 cup chopped onion
2 teaspoons minced garlic
2 cups fat-free vegetarian ground meat
2 teaspoons fat-free spaghetti sauce

Steam or microwave hot dogs. Put hot dogs in buns. Sauté onion and garlic. Add ground meat and cook 5 minutes. Then add spaghetti sauce. Cook 10 minutes on low heat and serve a large spoonful on each hot dog.

Pizza Ivan 2

Serves 4

Per Serving

Calories   275
Fat grams   2

1/2 cup lukewarm water
1 teaspoon yeast
1 teaspoon honey
1 teaspoon olive oil
1 teaspoon herbs
1/2 teaspoon salt
1/2 teaspoon pepper
1 1/2 cups all-purpose flour
1/2 cup semolina
1/2 cup cornmeal
1 cup spaghetti sauce
12 ounces fat-free ham, sliced
12 ounces fat-free shredded cheese

Preheat oven to 300°. Dissolve yeast in water. Add honey and oil until blended (use electric mixer). Combine herbs and sift with flour, semolina, and cornmeal, being careful not to oversift. Cover and refrigerate until double in size. Remove from refrigerator, knead, and form into two balls. Cover and let dough rise again. Sprinkle flour on table and roll balls with a roller until round. Heat cookie sheet in oven. Bake 15 minutes or until dough rises. Remove from oven and top with tomato sauce, ham, and cheese. Bake 8 to 10 minutes more, or freeze up to 1 week before baking.

Mexican Food

Cheese Enchiladas

2 tomatoes
1/2 onion
1 clove garlic
1 teaspoon cumin
Nonfat, nonstick spray
1 pound spinach
12 corn tortillas
1 pound fat-free cheese
1/2 cup cream

Serves 4

Per Serving
Calories   450
Fat grams   1

Puree tomatoes, onion, garlic, and cumin. Bring to boil. Spray skillet with nonfat, nonstick spray. Cook spinach until tender. Heat tortillas by placing in skillet for a few seconds. Roll tortilla with cheese and sauce. Put three on each plate and cover with sauce. Garnish with a little cream.

Turkey Fajitas

1 can fat-free refried beans
1 onion, sliced
1 green pepper, sliced
1 tomato, diced
1 fat-free smoked turkey breast, cut into strips
8 fat-free wheat tortillas
1/2 cup salsa
1/2 cup fat-free cream

Serves 4

Per Serving
Calories   410
Fat grams   3

Heat refried beans. Sauté onion and pepper until tender. Add tomato and turkey. Warm tortillas, fill them with turkey, and roll up. Serve with salsa, a spoonful of cream, and beans on the side.

Ham and Cheese Burritos

Serves 4

Per Serving

Calories   420
Fat grams   3

1/2 onion, diced
1 green pepper, diced
1 tomato, diced
8 fat-free wheat tortillas
8 fat-free cheese slices
8 fat-free ham slices
4 avocado slices
1/2 cup fat-free cream

Combine in a bowl onion, green pepper, and tomato. Put a slice of cheese and a slice of ham on each tortilla and bake in oven 350° for 5 minutes. Cut in 4 pieces and serve garnished with avocado and cream. Serve with tomato mixture on the side.

Tinga Chicken Tostada

Serves 4

Per Serving

Calories   400
Fat grams   1

4 chicken breasts, without skin
1 teaspoon minced garlic
1 onion, sliced
2 cups fat-free spaghetti sauce
8 corn tortillas
1 can fat-free refried beans
1/2 cup fat-free cream
1 cup chopped lettuce

Cook chicken breasts and shred them. Sauté garlic and onion until tender. Add spaghetti sauce and shredded chicken. Toast tortillas in microwave 6 minutes or until crisp. Heat beans and spread on tortillas with chicken. Top with cream and lettuce. Serve immediately.

Pasta

Stuffed Cannellonis with Spinach

1 cup spaghetti sauce
8 fat-free slices bacon
Nonfat, nonstick spray
1 teaspoon minced garlic
2 bags spinach
1 teaspoon herbs
1 bag cannellonis
2 teaspoons fat-free parmesan cheese

Serves 4

Per Serving
Calories   290
Fat grams   3

Heat spaghetti sauce. Sauté bacon and crumble finely. Spray skillet with nonfat, nonstick spray and sauté garlic, spinach, and herbs. When spinach is cooked, mix with bacon and fill cannellonis. Serve topped with spaghetti sauce and parmesan cheese.

Spaghetti Bolognese

Serves 4

Per Serving

Calories   350
Fat grams   2

12 ounces spaghetti
butter spray
Nonfat, nonstick spray
2 teaspoons minced garlic
1/2 cup chopped onion
1 pound fat-free vegetarian ground meat
2 teaspoons herbs
2 teaspoons Sauce Fifth Avenue
1 26-ounce jar fat-free pasta sauce
1 cup fat-free parmesan cheese
1/2 cup fat-free butter

Cook spaghetti, rinse, and drain. In a bowl mix with a little butter spray. Spray skillet with nonfat, nonstick spray and sauté garlic and onion until dark red. Add meat and season with herbs and Sauce Fifth Avenue. Cook on low heat 10 minutes. Just before serving, reheat pasta by boiling 1 minute or, in microwave, heat pasta with 1 cup sauce and 2 teaspoons parmesan cheese on top.

Vegetable Lasagna

1 16-ounce package lasagna
1 zucchini, diced
1 squash, diced
2 cups sliced mushrooms
1 eggplant, diced
2 teaspoons herbs
2 teaspoons Sauce Fifth Avenue
2 teaspoons garlic powder
Nonfat, nonstick spray
4 cups fat-free grated cheese
1 26-ounce jar fat-free pasta sauce

Serves 4

Per Serving
Calories   425
Fat grams   2

Cook pasta, rinse with cold water, and drain. Steam vegetables. Put in a bowl and season with herbs, Sauce Fifth Avenue, and garlic. Spray lasagna pan with nonfat, nonstick spray and place one layer of lasagna noodles on bottom, then layer of vegetables, then layer of cheese, then sauce. Repeat until ingredients are gone. Cover with aluminum foil and bake at 300° for 20 minutes.

Seven Seas Linguini

Serves 4

Per Serving

Calories   450
Fat grams   5

12 ounces linguini
1 cup fat-free butter
Nonfat, nonstick spray
2 teaspoons minced garlic
1/2 cup chopped onion
12 ounces scallops
12 ounces shrimp, shelled and deveined
12 ounces catfish
12 ounces salmon
12 ounces crab
3 teaspoons herbs
3 teaspoons Sauce Fifth Avenue
4 cups fat-free milk
1 can fat-free evaporated milk
4 teaspoons garlic powder
3 teaspoons cornstarch

Cook linguini, rinse with cold water, and drain. Put in a bowl and mix with a little butter. Spray skillet with non-fat, nonstick spray. Sauté garlic and onion. Add all seafood, herbs, and Sauce Fifth Avenue. In a saucepan, boil milk and evaporated milk on low heat. Add garlic powder. Mix cornstarch in 1 cup lukewarm water and stir into milk until thickened. Serve pasta topped with seafood, sauce, and parmesan cheese, if desired.

Drinks

Varsdero Punch

10 ounces fresh pineapple
1 banana
1 cup shredded coconut
2 teaspoons artificial rum flavoring
1 pound ice
2 teaspoons sugar or 1 envelope noncaloric sugar
   substitute

Serves 2

Per Serving
Calories   210
Fat grams   2

Clean pineapple and cut into pieces. Puree all ingredients in blender except a few pineapple wedges. Serve immediately in a glass, garnished with a pineapple triangle.

Good Morning Juice

12 ounces papaya
4 cups orange juice
1/2 cup sugar or 2 envelopes noncaloric sugar
   substitute
1/2 pound ice
1 teaspoon lemon juice

Serves 2

Per Serving
Calories   200
Fat grams   0

Clean papaya. Puree in blender with other ingredients. Drink within 5 minutes of preparation to receive full nutritional value.

Watermelon Juice

Serves 6

24 ounces watermelon
2 quarts cold water
2 teaspoons lemon juice
1 pound ice in cubes
1 cup sugar or 4 envelopes noncaloric sugar substitute

Per Serving

Calories   80
Fat grams   0

Dice one-half watermelon. Puree other half watermelon with water, lemon, sugar, and 1/2 pound ice. Pour in a pitcher with remaining ice and diced watermelon. Refrigerate before serving.

Desserts

Carrot Cake

1 cup all-purpose flour
1 cup wheat flour
2 teaspoons baking soda
1 teaspoon baking powder
2 teaspoons cinnamon
1/2 teaspoon nutmeg
6 egg whites
1 1/2 cups sugar
1/2 cup fat-free buttermilk
1 teaspoon vanilla
1 cup applesauce
2 cups shredded carrots
1/2 cup raisins
Nonfat, nonstick spray

Meringue:
8 ounces fat-free
  cream cheese
8 ounces marsh-
  mallow cream
1 teaspoon lemon
  juice
1/2 teaspoon vanilla

Serves 12

Per Serving
Calories   360
Fat grams   1

Combine flours, baking soda, baking powder, cinnamon, and nutmeg in a bowl. In another bowl beat egg whites on high speed until stiff. Add sugar, then gradually add buttermilk, vanilla, and applesauce. Fold in flour mixture slowly. Add carrots and raisins. Spray casserole dish with nonfat, nonstick spray. Pour mixture into it and bake at 350° for 35 to 40 minutes or until a toothpick comes out clean when inserted in the middle. Meringue: Combine all ingredients and pour over cake when cool.

Cheesecake

Serves 12

Per Serving

Calories   400
Fat grams   3

24 ounces fat-free cream cheese, room temperature
1 cup sugar
1 teaspoon vanilla
Nonfat, nonstick spray
1 cup graham cracker crumbs

Meringue:
6 egg whites
16 ounces fat-free cream
3 teaspoons sugar
1 teaspoon vanilla

Combine and beat on low speed cream cheese, sugar, and vanilla. Be careful not to beat too long. Spray pie plate with nonfat, nonstick spray and press graham cracker crumbs into a crust. Pour in cream cheese mixture. Bake at 325° for 45 minutes or until pie is puffed up in the middle. Meringue: Beat egg whites until stiff. Combine cream, sugar, and vanilla and fold into egg whites. Pour on pie and bake 5 to 7 minutes. Let pie cool, then refrigerate for at least 2 hours before serving.

Strawberry Yogurt

Serves 2

Per Serving

Calories   210
Fat grams   0

8 strawberries
3 cups skim milk
3 cups fat-free vanilla yogurt
1 teaspoon vanilla
1 teaspoon artificial rum flavoring
2 envelopes noncaloric sugar substitute
1 teaspoon cinnamon

In blender combine all ingredients but two strawberries and cinnamon. Serve in a glass topped with 1 strawberry and sprinkled with cinnamon.

Cuban Yogurt

1 cup skim milk
1 shot espresso coffee
2 teaspoons sugar or 1 envelope noncaloric sugar
   substitute
2 teaspoons fat-free chocolate syrup
6 cups fat-free vanilla yogurt
1 teaspoon cinnamon

Serves 2

Per Serving
Calories   300
Fat grams   0

In blender combine milk, espresso coffee, and sugar or noncaloric sugar substitute. Blend in chocolate syrup and yogurt on maximum speed till foam appears. Serve sprinkled with cinnamon on top.

Strawberry Parfait

8 whole strawberries
2 teaspoons vanilla
2 teaspoons artificial rum flavoring
2 cans fat-free condensed milk
32 strawberries cut in half
1 cup fat-free whipped cream
1 teaspoon cinnamon

Serves 4

Per Serving
Calories   320
Fat grams   0

Puree 8 strawberries. Add vanilla, rum, and condensed milk. Refrigerate at least 3 hours. Fill glass half full of strawberries cut in half. Add strawberry mixture and top with whipped cream and cinnamon.

Rice Pudding

Serves 4

Per Serving
Calories 300
Fat grams 1

2 sticks of cinnamon
1 orange peel
5 cups water
2 cups white rice
4 cups skim milk
1 can fat-free condensed milk
1/2 cup raisins
2 teaspoons vanilla
1 teaspoon cinnamon

Boil cinnamon sticks and orange peel in water. Add rice and cook on low heat until rice is tender. Remove cinnamon sticks and orange peel if you like. Combine condensed milk, raisins, and vanilla in saucepan. Add rice and stir over low heat until mixture comes to a slow boil. Serve in glasses. Top with cinnamon.

Coffee Caramel

Serves 4

Per Serving
Calories 260
Fat grams 0

1/2 cup sugar
1 12-ounce package fat-free Philadelphia cream cheese
1 cup skim milk
1 cup fat-free condensed milk
1 cup egg beaters
2 teaspoons coffee, brewed

Heat sugar in a glass loaf pan until caramelized. Cover the walls of the pan with the caramel and let cool. Puree cream cheese, milk, condensed milk, egg, and coffee. Pour into loaf pan and cover with aluminum foil. Set in larger pan, which is filled with 1 inch water. Cover both pans with aluminum foil. Cook on stove with water at low boil approximately 1 hour or until toothpick comes out clean after inserting in the middle. Check water level periodically to make certain it doesn't all evaporate. Cool and remove from pan.

Pineapple Upside-Down Cake

2 cups applesauce
1/2 cup sugar
1 cup egg beaters
1 can fat-free condensed milk
3 cups all-purpose flour
1 teaspoon baking powder
1 cup pineapple juice
Nonfat, nonstick spray
1/2 cup brown sugar
8 pineapple slices in juice
8 cherries

Serves 8

Per Serving

Calories	300
Fat grams	1

Combine in a bowl applesauce, sugar, egg, and condensed milk. Sift flour with baking powder and fold into mixture. Gently stir in pineapple juice. Grease pan with nonfat, nonstick spray and cover with brown sugar. Arrange pineapple slices and place cherries in the holes. Pour apple mixture over pineapples. Bake 45 minutes to 1 hour at 350°. Immediately after baking, turn pan over onto serving platter and take cake from pan.

Strawberry Biscuit

1/2 cup egg beaters
4 cups fat-free pancake flour
3 teaspoons noncaloric sugar substitute
2 cups skim milk
1 cup strawberries
1 cup fat-free condensed milk
1 teaspoon vanilla
3 cups sliced strawberries
1 cup fat-free plain yogurt

Serves 4

Per Serving

Calories	300
Fat grams	2

Mix in a bowl egg, flour, and noncaloric sugar substitute. Add milk until thick enough to make into balls the size of golf balls. Bake at 350° for 20 minutes. In blender combine strawberries, condensed milk, and vanilla. Mix sliced strawberries with yogurt. Cut biscuits and fill them with strawberries and yogurt mixture. Serve topped with condensed milk mixture.

Banana Pudding

Serves 4

Per Serving

Calories 400
Fat grams 3

4 teaspoons cornstarch
1 cup cold water
5 cups skim milk
10 envelopes noncaloric sugar substitute
2 teaspoons vanilla
2 teaspoons artificial banana flavoring
1 teaspoon artificial coconut flavoring
Nonfat, nonstick spray
4 sliced bananas
1 box vanilla wafers

Mix cornstarch in 1 cup cold water. Bring to boil milk, sugar substitute, vanilla, banana flavoring, and coconut flavoring. Slowly stir in cornstarch mixture until a pudding consistency is reached. Spray pan lightly and alternate wafers, banana slices, wafers, and pudding until full. Refrigerate at least 3 hours and serve cold.

To have a life-changing experience, I encourage you to act on the truths in this book. For this reason, I have also published a Workbook that goes with it. Please consider giving it to yourself as a gift to help you put into practice what you have learned. To help you right now, I have provided the following pages to help you get started.

What Is My Motivation to Lose Weight?

(You may have many)

_____

_____

_____

_____

_____

_____

_____

_____

_____

What Are the Things I Want to Do

When I Reach My Ideal Weight?

_____

_____

_____

_____

_____

_____

_____

_____

_____

Other Books by T. D. Jakes

Lay Aside the Weight (Workbook)
So You Call Yourself a Man!
Woman, Thou Art Loosed! (Hardcover)
Woman, Thou Art Loosed! (Devotional)
Loose That Man and Let Him Go! (Hardcover)
Loose That Man and Let Him Go! (Softcover)
Loose That Man and Let Him Go! (Workbook)
T. D. Jakes Speaks to Men!
T. D. Jakes Speaks to Women!
Woman, Thou Art Loosed (Spanish)
Loose That Man and Let Him Go! (Spanish)
T. D. Jakes Speaks to Men! (Spanish)
T. D. Jakes Speaks to Women! (Spanish)

To contact T. D. Jakes, write:

T. D. Jakes Ministries
P. O. Box 210887
Dallas, Texas 75211

Additional copies of this book
and other book titles from ALBURY PUBLISHING
are available at your local bookstore.

In Canada, books are available from:

Word Alive
P. O. Box 670
Niverville, Manitoba
CANADA ROA 1BO

ALBURY PUBLISHING
P. O. Box 470406
Tulsa, Oklahoma 74147-0406